CANNABIS COOKBOOK

Easy to Follow Recipe Guide for Candy, Ice-cream, Muffins, Cookies, Brownies & So Much More! Extract Your Own CBD and make edible THC-infused and Irresistible Recipes.

MARY CERVANTES

Table of Contents

INTRODUCTION

The normal responses one gets from referencing or saying the word "Cannabis" are " Do you smoke?" or "would I be able to get a hit of your joint?" This is because of the awful notoriety that has been connected to this herb because of stigmatization and criticism. In this case, if you could permit yourself to move past, at that point, will you have the option to get the genuine advantages of this great herb.

Let's be honest, regardless of whether you need to call it "marijuana", "cannabis" or even "weed", there is no denying that this comes with an exceptional number of therapeutic purposes and obviously, is an extraordinary source of resisting the urge to panic. One the most ideal ways you can accomplish this is by preparing and utilizing it to make meals. Of course! You can cook pretty much anything with cannabis and in spite of mainstream thinking it isn't hard in any way.

These pre-made, pre-bundled cannabis mixed treats are more open to various persons especially patients these days than any time in recent, yet tragically, numerous edibles, despite everything come pressed with sugar, high fructose corn syrup, and other undesirable ingredients. While these foods which are already processed can be a simple method to get cured in a hurry, numerous individuals and clinical cannabis patients incline toward making their own medicated snacks and meals already infused and in light of current circumstances.

The restorative characteristics of this plant follow back through written history. Old civic establishments, including China, Greece, India, and medieval societies archived cannabis just like a helpful treatment for people and even creatures. It was an exceptionally normal treatment all through the eighteenth and nineteenth centuries in America. Cannabis was the doctors' essential agony reliever until the disclosure of ibuprofen. Cannabis was an unmistakable piece of the US Pharmacopeia until 1942, and a few significant pharmaceutical organizations appropriated it and held licenses for medications containing cannabis.

It was prohibited by the Marijuana Tax Act of 1937 and less ordinarily utilized from that point. In 1996 California voters passed Proposition 215, which was the main state law to permit patients a lawful option to utilize medical cannabis. From that point forward, numerous different states have passed comparative enactment by voter activity or the administrative procedure. In 2009 the US Congress lifted a boycott, permitting Washington DC occupants lawful access to medical cannabis.

As of now a few nations, including the Netherlands, Canada, Spain, and Italy permit cannabis to be recommended in its plant structure. The American Medical Association (AMA) and the American College of Physicians (ACP), the world's biggest associations of doctors, have required the rescheduling of cannabis studies to investigate its health advantages. Clinical associations over the globe have embraced the health advantages of cannabis, and it is indeed developing as a genuine treatment in clinical circles.

California and different states have cannabis apportioning aggregates, or dispensaries, where patients can get to their meds in a perfect and safe condition. Patients keep on increasing safe access to these meds while clinical experts, patient activists, and concerned keep on separating the hindrances of many years of falsehood, and permit reality with regards to the advantages of cannabis to become well known. Legitimate, political, and social changes keep on advancing inside the clinical cannabis scene.

Antiquated individuals only ate their cannabis, sparing seeds for food, and utilizing the resinous blossoms for therapeutic, recreational, and otherworldly use. Probably the most seasoned formula for cannabis infused food comes to us from India. In the Western world, cannabis tinctures, which break down the plant's dynamic ingredients into a solution of alcohol, would remain broadly accessible in drug stores until the late 1800s, offered over the counter as a treatment for depression, pain, stomach cramps, and other basic ailments.

However, the idea of smoking cannabis didn't get stylish in the United States until from the get-go in the twentieth century, while relocating Mexican laborers acquainted the training with the Southwest, and voyaging jazz performers hence spread it to the remainder of the landmass. So, while smoking this herb flaunts a long and great family in the cutting-edge world, always remember that eating cannabis is a blessed human custom that is actually more seasoned than history.

Understanding Cannabis sativa as essentially another feeding, recuperating, accommodating bloom is critical to expelling a significant part of the fear and misjudging, piled upon a hapless public and to a great extent, an innocuous plant by many years of government purposeful publicity. Cannabis brownies, a backbone of counterculture food since the 1950s, remain the most widely recognized way current individuals initially ingest cannabis.

During the early periods, the food revolution turned into a piece of the general countercultural way of life, as nonconformists went veggie lover and explored ethnic foods which were then unbelievable in the United States, for example, tofu and seaweed, falafel and hummus, curries and lentils, burritos and arepas. More than anything, they looked for something bona fide to eat in a nation rapidly giving up its culinary legacy for inexpensive food and plastic-wrapped, solidified, prepackaged TV suppers.

Keeping in mind that the unfair generalization of stoners as shoddy foods addicts endures right up 'til today, the reality remains that counterculture cooking advocated by cannabis-cherishing nonconformists and health foodies has given an equal food movement dependent on great sustenance and natural cultivating processes that our undeniably unhealthy society woefully needs. To be sure, the development of the local food movement and grasp of occasional, economical cooking by food specialists across the country owes its underlying foundations to a hippie reasonableness that is green in all faculties of the word.

In 1996, the memorable entry of California's Proposition 215 successfully sanctioned clinical cannabis in California, opening the entryway for an ever increasing number of individuals to understand the advantages of eating their stash as opposed to smoking it, which incorporate protecting the strength of the respiratory framework, diminishing the smell of cannabis smoke on all hands and clothing, and the capacity to watchfully medicate in numerous spots where smoking would be unseemly—also unlawful. Cannabis additionally delivers various impacts when ingested through the digestive system, instead of consumed by the lungs, with most clients revealing a more drawn out enduring experience that gives a high to both the body and brain.

Today, there is a vastly improved comprehension of cannabis and the mending parts these plants have. Numerous examinations have demonstrated exactly how amazing this healing plant can be. Present day research gives suggestions that cannabis, when ingested, is an important guide in the treatment of a wide scope of conditions. These include relief from pain– especially that caused from nerve harm – queasiness, spasticity, glaucoma, and movement issues. Cannabis is additionally an amazing stimulant for appetite, explicitly for patients suffering from HIV, AIDS, or dementia. Rising studies recommends that cannabis' therapeutic properties may even secure one against certain kinds of threatening tumors, and go about as a neuroprotective.

As a whole plant, Cannabis is amazingly versatile as an ingredient. Of late, the clinical cannabis "edibles" industry has been the way to moving past brownies, extending our cannabis palates cosmically, as creative and highly imaginative canna-culinary specialists in a now serious field have injected the herb into pretty much any dish you can envision.

You can discover prepared, herb-mixed plate of mixed greens dressings, exquisite plunges, powdered beverages, soft drinks, smoothies, baked products, and desserts in numerous dispensaries, also topical moisturizers, rub oils, and cleansers utilizing cannabis as a functioning recuperating ingredient. All in all, what does the sanctioning of recreational cannabis mean for food researchers? As cannabis becomes legalized, a few organizations have bounced on the chance to create "edibles", or food items that pass on the impacts of cannabis in a consumable, as opposed to a smoke form. Cannabis clients have since quite a while ago made their own natively constructed edibles (the most widely recognized model being pot brownies), yet by making it themselves, those clients had the option to tailor the measure of the cannabis extricate, just as control who expends their item.

Offering a delectable option in contrast to smoking or disintegrating cannabis, cannabis edibles are food and refreshment items that have been implanted with cannabis. Shoppers who appreciate cannabis edibles ordinarily lean toward the all-encompassing and progressively extraordinary impacts that they offer contrasted with different sorts of cannabis items. A wide range of kinds of cannabis edibles are accessible to buy in legitimate cannabis states all through the United States, where the greater part of the states have legalized recreational or clinical cannabis. It's additionally regular now for cannabis epicureans to make their own cannabis implanted food at home. While cannabis edibles are well known among standard, long haul cannabis clients, they're additionally a supported decision among beginners who are being acquainted with cannabis for the absolute first time and are searching for a simple method to take their cannabis.

With all the choices accessible to clinical cannabis patients today, many are deciding to investigate strategies for curing past the conventional pipe or paper. Products or items infused with cannabis, ordinarily alluded to as edibles, give another choice to patients who can't, or decide not to smoke their cannabis. Edibles come in a wide range of assortments including brownies, candy, chocolate bars, cookies, drinks, pills, snacks, spreads and that's only the tip of the iceberg. There are even a few organizations that offer a "medicated" meals on-wheels administration for patients that can't genuinely go out.

Cannabis consumed orally enters the circulatory system in the wake of being processed or separated in the stomach and is absorbed in the digestive organs. Eating items or products already infused is a more beneficial option in contrast to breathing in cannabis smoke in light of the fact that there is no presentation to carbon, tar, carcinogens or cancer-causing agents, and so forth.

Ideally, as cannabis gets well known as basically another culinary herb, there will be expanded appreciation for its one of a kind flavor profile and stop endeavoring to conceal it. Figuring out how to cook with and share cannabis is an extraordinary blessing—engaging, edifying, elevating—and one that must be shared. Recipes in this cookbook have been consolidated in light of the fact that it has been seen that cannabis work wonders on several people and different activities are being carried out to guarantee that each and every individual who needs them has these tools.

CHAPTER ONE: INSIGHT INTO THE WORLD OF CANNABIS

Cannabis (stick like) sativa (planted or sown) is a yearly plant with long, toothy leaves and flowers which contains trichomes, hairs secured with resin glands which are sticky and in the form of crystals. The flowers sprout on branches from a woody focal stalk that develops from one-foot-high to twenty feet high. These trees can be discovered developing under circle houses along Colorado's ripe Western Slope and in northern California.

Cannabis, otherwise called marijuana among different names, is a psychoactive medication from the Cannabis plant utilized essentially for clinical or recreational purposes. The fundamental psychoactive part of cannabis is tetrahydrocannabinol (THC), which is one of the 483 known ingredients in the plant, including in any event 65 different cannabinoids. Cannabis can be utilized by smoking, vaporizing, inside food, or as a concentrate.

Cannabis is generally utilized recreationally or as a therapeutic medication, despite the fact that it might likewise be utilized for other spiritual or worldly purposes. In 2013, somewhere in the range of 128 and 232 million individuals utilized cannabis (2.7% to 4.9% of the worldwide populace between the ages of 15 and 65). It is the most regularly utilized illicit medication both on the planet and the United States, however it is likewise legal in certain wards. The nations with the most noteworthy use among grown-ups starting at 2018 are Zambia, the United States, Canada, and Nigeria.

In 2016, 51% of individuals in the United States had utilized cannabis in the course of their lives. About 12% had utilized it in the previous year, and 7.3% had utilized it in the previous month.

While cannabis plants have been cultivated since the 3rd millennium BCE, some evidence proposes that it was being smoked for psychoactive impacts at any rate 2,500 years prior. Since the mid twentieth century, cannabis has been dependent upon lawful limitations.

The ownership, use, and growing of cannabis is unlawful in many nations of the world. In 2013, Uruguay turned into the principal nation to authorize recreational utilization of cannabis. Different nations to do so are Canada, Georgia, and South Africa, alongside 11 states and the District of Columbia in the United States (however the medication remains governmentally unlawful). Utilization of cannabis medically, requiring the endorsement of a doctor, has been sanctioned in a more prominent number of nations.

Cannabis develops from seeds in living soil, delivering leaves and flowers from sun and downpour. Leaves from the cannabis plant are splendid green and have a particular shape with five or seven flyers. The blooming tops and upper leaves are canvassed in a clingy sap. For a large number of years, the cannabis plant developed wild and free, on high fields and peaks, in chasms and fields. The early people found and sustained it, and this gave individuals fiber and medication for a considerable length of time.

CLASSIFICATIONS OF THE CANNABIS PLANT

Cannabis comes in three classifications, each with its own particular character. Sativa and Indica are generally normal.

- Cannabis sativa is tall and slim, with long, thin, pointy leaves and fleecy, fruity flowers. When eaten, it conveys a splendid, overwhelming euphoria that numerous individuals acknowledge for daytime use.

  Cannabis sativa L, or hemp, is a non-psychoactive cannabis subspecies utilized fundamentally for food and fiber. It gives important supplements and different advantages to people; however it won't get anybody high, regardless of the amount eaten. Industrial form of hemp is reproduced for fiber, food, and fuel as opposed to flowers, which is the place THC is found, and hemp contains just about 0.25 percent of the psychoactive cannabinoids.

  This recently rising clinical cannabis edibles industry is an ongoing marvel, however food made with hemp and body-care items have been a backbone in numerous health food stores for a considerable length of time. Hemp and cannabis are connected plants however, extraordinary in a couple of significant ways. Hemp contains next to zero detectable THC; thus, it isn't psychoactive in any structure.

Yet, while hemp inherently comes up short on the synthetics that make people euphoric, it despite everything, contains numerous fortifying amino acids and antioxidants. Hemp likewise contains cannabidiol (CBD), a significant cannabinoid with numerous therapeutic impacts. Hemp flour, oil, protein powder, seeds, and milk are staples of a healthy eating regimen. Normal food organizations have begun utilizing hemp seeds and flour in solidified waffles, granola bars, breakfast oat, and other food products.

Hemp can likewise be found as an ingredient in numerous soaps and cleansers, moisturizers, and emollients, while the strands of the plant make solid paper and materials. Despite the fact that hemp is the calm plant cousin to cannabis, growing a hemp crop in the United States is as yet unlawful because of the misinformed war on cannabis, thus America keeps on bringing in hemp from Canada and China to use for food and clothes.

- Cannabis Indica is low and thick, with wide and well round leaves and more tightly structure. When eaten, it conveys a comfortable, calming, loosened up all-over body impact.

- Cannabis ruderalis is less fiery than Indica and sativa, developing just around two feet tall, and is utilized for the most part in crossbreeding for its capacity to blossom without changes in light cycles. A great many people don't devour it since it doesn't contain a lot of THC.

COMPONENTS OF THE CANNABIS PLANT

Cannabinoids

The cannabis plant contains dynamic chemical compounds called cannabinoids, which are something of a supernatural occurrence. In 1988, researchers found that the crystal-like hairs containing resin glands, or trichomes, on cannabis leaves and flowers, contain active compounds of chemical nature (almost ninety have been isolated up until this point) which plug into cannabinoid receptors in the brain. These plant-based forms of chemicals that is produced by our brains when under pressure—a duplicate of the cannabinoids in human breast milk—convey incredible antioxidants and can move neurological and physiological patterns. Different plants, for example, cacao, dark pepper, echinacea, and turmeric convey cannabinoids, yet none are as productive and amazing as those in the cannabis plant. In 2003, the government was conceded US Patent 6,630,507 for the utilization of cannabinoids as antioxidant agents and neuroprotectants.

They're being examined as medicines for Alzheimer's ailment, Parkinson's sickness, PTSD, and stroke patients. THC, the most renowned—and supported—cannabinoid in cannabis is delta-9terahydrocannabinol, or THC. THC triggers CB1 receptors, which are likewise mediated by anandamide, the main human cannabinoid discovered in 1992. CB1 receptors decide how we see, smell, listen, and feel appetite, joy, and pain—which is the reason everything is wonderful, food tastes and scents astonishing, and reality television can be pleasant when individuals eat cannabis. THC additionally actuates CB2 receptors in the liver, heart, kidneys, veins, endocrine organs, and lymph cells, making it a decent tonic, yet its psychoactive component has made it lovable component among cannabis clients.

CBD

Cannabidiol (CBD) is an exceptional cannabinoid that is getting elevated level consideration since it conveys health advantages without getting patients high. CBD doesn't bind to CB1 receptors, where psychoactive effects are activated, and can really stop the THC's psychoactive effects by contradicting its activities at CB1 receptors. The CBD cannabinoid stimulates receptors that mediate pain, irritation, and internal heat level and direct oxygen, blood, and dopamine. CBD hinders serotonin receptor signals, giving it an upper impact. It's being read as a treatment for individuals with nervousness, rest and dietary problems, pain, and being nauseous.

Terpenes

Cannabis gets its extraordinary smell and flavor (normally alluded to as "damp" or "loud") from in excess of 120 terpenes, pungent oils created in the trichomes to entice pollinators and shoo away predators and sicknesses. Every single fragrant plant, for example, pine and citrus have terpenes, yet cannabis has more than other plants. When cannabis flowers are dried and cured, oxidation changes over terpenes into terpenoids, which associate with cannabinoids in the human body to balance the impacts of THC and control dopamine and serotonin.

HOW IT GROWS

One of mankind's most seasoned agricultural yields, cannabis develops in around four or five months in many atmospheres. It's as simple to grow (or as troublesome, contingent upon your planting skills) as tomatoes. Like all plants, cannabis reacts best to a little nurture and great conditions: all around circulated air through, mineral-rich soil also with nutrients; clean water; and southern exposure with great daylight.

Cannabis adjusts to not exactly perfect conditions, as cultivators constrained into woods and alleys all through preclusion can authenticate, yet it prefers the pinch of a green thumb. Much the same as tomatoes and roses, cannabis can be pruned and prepared for better yield, and it prefers sustained, well amended soil, a stake or cage to incline toward, and a nursery for warmth protection (still an issue, even where cannabis is legal).

The greatest distinction among cannabis and most different plants in the nursery is that it's dioecious, which means each seed is male or female. Male plants produce less gum and can blossom prior so they can fertilize females and afterward, crucial, gradually wilt. They wallop the young ladies with pollen, given the opportunity, making the young female plants dreary and seedy.

Consequently, most planters yank the young male plants when they show erect little bloom balls. The seedless, single young female plants produce more resins with higher amounts of delta-9-tetrahydrocannabinol (THCP), the cannabinoid that gets individuals high, and become known as sinsemilla. Cannabis plants cultivated from clones, or cuttings from plants that are matured, are for the most part females, so this procedure isn't vital.)

PROCESSING CANNABIS

Cannabis producers have the same number of various methods for processing and handling the plant as the plant has cultivars. Each planter or farmer depends on their own technique, and they all spread shared opinion. Cannabis ought to be dried and cured so it holds enough dampness to use however, is sufficiently dry to forestall molds. Appropriate restoring, which is reliant on the plant's hereditary qualities and condition, upgrades and preserves the plant's fragrance, flavor, and strength and expels chlorophyll. Chlorophyll gives cannabis the solid "green" taste that turns numerous individuals off yet additionally gives important supplements when ingested.

In general, cannabis plants are prepared to be harvested when the trichomes (clingy resin found on the flowers) turn shady white or light golden and the leaves begin blurring and take on autumn tints (a characteristic procedure called senescence). Plants can be gathered in stages, starting from the top, so less develop blossoms on the lower portion of the plant can have an additional week or so in the sun. Cannabis ought to be collected in the first part of the day in light of the fact that specific terpenes vanish in heat as the day heats up. When the plants are collected, the fan leaves are expelled for squeezing, cooking, fertilizing the soil, or mulching. Previously, thought about as a waste item, these leaves are at long last getting praises for their non-psychoactive medical advantages.

The plants or individual branches are hung topsy turvy on clotheslines or spread out on a screen to dry for four to ten days, contingent upon the atmosphere and planned use. For the smoothest flavor, cannabis ought to be dried as gradually as possible in a sixty-to seventy-degree room (dampness and warmth support shape) with great wind current that is not blowing straightforwardly on the plants. Fans, radiators, and dehumidifiers are some of the time important to keep up temperature and humidity. For little reaps, containers of water or wet towels in the drying room can be sufficient to keep up the dampness. At the point when the stems are practically hard enough to snap off however, the blossoms are not yet brittle, the plants are prepared to trim and cure. Cutting is the way toward clipping off the little sugar leaves encompassing the flowers, which can be spared and utilized for cooking and tinctures. Trimming cuts out the blossoms' nectar, where the vast majority of the sticky trichomes, rich with cannabinoids, dwell.

STORAGE OF CANNABIS

Classic, Ball or Mason containers with hermetically sealed tops, are a great many people's vessel of choice for cannabis stockpiling. The jar should be given a decent wash and store cannabis away from heat, light, dampness, and wind stream. Cannabis should save for a year or more in a container with a decent seal. Cannabis can likewise be put away in a water/air proof wooden box, and a few organizations showcase curing and storing boxes like humidors for stogies. The Cannador, a designer box that keeps up perfect dampness for cannabis stockpiling, sells for two or three hundred dollars.

BUYER'S GUIDE

Today, individuals with specialist's suggestions and grown-ups in states where cannabis is legitimate can pick cannabis cultivars like they pick varietals of wine, whiskey, espresso, cheddar, and chocolate. They can analyze and purchase (at no little cost) high quality sinsemilla to improve their state of mind, help them rest, and add the correct spice to stew, browsing handfuls if not several cultivars with names like Afghan Kush, Blue Dream, Cheese, Girl Scout Cookies, and Pineapple Kush in each flavor from mint, chocolate, and musk to fruit, spices, and berries. They can choose sativas for daytime use, indicas for rest, and any number of sweet cultivars for making cake—and that is before they go to the racks loaded with bubble hash, wax, shatter, oils, edibles, drinks, capsules, tinctures, teas, moisturizers, and sexual oils. For help with each one of those decisions, they can go to a "budtender" or "cannabarista".

DISPENSARIES AND RETAIL STORES

Strolling into a dispensary or retail location just because is celebratory for a few, overpowering for other people. For long-lasting cannabis clients, seeing containers loaded with manicured flowers, for lawful deal in a retail foundation, is dreamlike. For clinical cannabis patients and others investigating cannabis for the first time (or the first run through in quite a while), seeing each one of those containers is befuddling.

Regardless of whether you're visiting a retail store in a state where cannabis is lawful or approach a dispensary, the first run through can be frightening. How would you realize where to purchase, what to purchase, and whether you're purchasing acceptable quality natural cannabis? What should cannabis smell like when the budtender opens the container and puts it right in front of you? What would it be advisable for it to resemble in the event that the budtender gives you an amplifying glass to look at it?

Where to Buy

Like coffee and alcohol stores, cannabis stores go from boutique to mega, with climates from crude to spa-like. A few dispensaries call themselves centers for wellness and offer cannabis notwithstanding massage, needle therapy, and other common treatments.) Customer administration agents (budtenders' legitimate industry name, however nobody considers them that) vary in information and presence also. How every foundation develops, gets, processes, and handles cannabis has a major effect in the nature of its products, particularly when you're purchasing natural cannabis. Do a little schoolwork.

At any rate, take a look at the site before you visit a cannabis dispensary. Discover to what extent they've been doing business. Do they guarantee to sell natural cannabis? Is it accurate to say that they are showcasing to individuals like you? Would you like to purchase your food and medication from a foundation that includes an ample "nurture" with a major green cannabis leaf on her chest in its ads?

The magnificence in the market of legal cannabis is that nobody needs to purchase cannabis from individuals they wouldn't ordinarily connect with any longer, and you'll realize immediately whether you're in the ideal spot. The primary thing you should see when you enter a dispensary is the mind-boggling smell of new cannabis. If you don't get hit with that aroma when you stroll in the entryway, that is a flag. The perfect aroma of good natural cannabis can't be contained, even in fixed glass containers. Most dispensaries and retail locations offer cannabis in three quality levels. In some cases, it is marked or color coded that way, however, pricing ordinarily reflects where a cultivar stands. All in all, cost reflects quality—much like wine.

The most effective method to Buy

Picking quality cannabis isn't too not quite the same as picking quality tomatoes. With natural cannabis, it's everything about scent and appearance—in a specific order. A similar decent sense that advises you not to purchase a tomato that is soft or smells musty will disclose to you when something's off about cannabis blossoms. In the event that cannabis smells like a bit of rotten bread, it may contain pathogens, for example, mold or parasite. In the event that it smells like nothing, you won't get the taste, fragrance, and experience you're after.

Quality natural cannabis is a healthy green, with traces of purple, orange, red, and red-orange hairs. Search for flowers shining with trichomes, the icing of crystal resin glands where cannabis' significant cannabinoids live. Trichome inclusion can be a decent sign of quality yet not generally the best marker of value hereditary qualities. The most ideal approach to discover is to follow your nose. The perfect, sharp smell of fragrant terpenes should hit you when the container is aired out. From that point,

fragrance is a profoundly personal inclination. Your nose will disclose to you when

you've hit the fragrant profile you're after. Trust it.

CHAPTER TWO: THE CANNABIS NATURE

GETTING THE MOST OUT OF IT

To determine the best and most affordable outcomes from cannabinated cooking, there should be remembrance of a few realities about the physical and chemical nature of cannabis and how it is broken down and assimilated in the digestive system. This is not to raise the trouble or perplexity in the complexities of science. However, a simple comprehension of certain subtleties will be of an incentive in settling on specific choices which will give the best outcomes for the least investment.

The Effect of Eating and Smoking Cannabis

The greatest distinction between eating cannabis and smoking it is the force and kind of high that occurs. Eating cannabis welcomes on an increasingly physical sensation, or "body high," which relieves sore muscles, relieves pain, helps in unwinding, and battles sleep deprivation, while giving feelings of warmth and tingling sensations. Edibles can likewise deliver an effectively hallucinogenic euphoria, which can last far longer than the run of the mill high from smoking.

Smoking is one of the numerous odd ceremonies of humankind. It is practiced all around, pretty much, in both crude and modern social orders. Huge numbers of individuals feel, that it isn't to the greatest advantage of our lungs to breathe in immense volumes of ashes. The warmth tars and cruel smoke from any material, be it tobacco, cannabis or delicate herb, bothers, meddles with oxygen consumption and may rush pneumonic disorders in people inclined to these. The coherent option in contrast to smoking cannabis is to ingest it.

Continuously remember that everybody's resistance is extraordinary, and people react to ingesting cannabis in various manners. Normally, one won't feel any outcomes following eating cannabis, since it should be processed to produce results, a procedure that can take somewhere in the range of thirty minutes to two hours relying upon the amount you ingest, and whether it's on a full or void stomach. So start with a little serving and don't eat any more cannabis food for in any event an hour, after the primary serving.

Smoking, as already established, is bothering to the throat and lungs. In the event that one is as of now a client of tobacco, such individual will at any rate be incurred to take in smoke. If an individual isn't a smoker, such person will most likely neglect to breathe in the cannabis smoke appropriately and in adequate volumes to accomplish the ideal state. The ingestion of grass is decadent instead of masochistic. Ingested in ordinary sums, there are no unsavory side effects. When eaten in exorbitant amounts, it might cause a slow inclination and ragged looking eyes the next day. At the point when cannabis is smoked, the impact is practically momentary.

A few supposed "creeper" grasses may take five minutes or so to come on totally, however a portion of the high is typically felt immediately. The high from smoking ordinarily endures from one to over two hours, and can be recovered when it is melting away by taking a couple of more tokes. At the point when cannabis is ingested, an individual must hold up thirty minutes to 90 minutes before the principal phases of the high are even taken note. After this, the euphoric state keeps on expanding. It might then last from four to eight hours, and now and again considerably more.

Those who've eaten an excessive amount of cannabis may feel panicky, restless, agoraphobic, disorganized, or very nearly an all-out "go nuts." Fear of "losing it completely" has additionally been accounted for. Should this transpire, retreat to a protected spot to rests, diminish the lights, inhale profoundly, drink a lot of liquids, eat non-cannabis food, and have yourself distracted by tuning in to your preferred music or viewing a film you like. Most presumably, you'll wind up snoozing, and in a couple of hours all the awkward feelings will have died down.

Solubility of Cannabis

THC, the substance active in cannabis isn't water soluble. It is dissolvable in oils, fats and alcohols. This has been known for a great many years. Recipes from certain nations, for example, India and other cannabis-eating human civilizations as a rule, necessitate that the cannabis be sauteed in margarine or a clarified butter known as "ghee" before mixing it with different ingredients. Lately, it is discovered that individuals boil and frequently steep the leaves, seeds and stems of cannabis in water and afterward drink cup after cup in quest for a high that may never show up. At that point they dispose of the leaves, which, however wet, are as yet still potent.

If the plant is of brilliant quality and has a lot of resin outwardly, it is conceivable, after arduous heating up, that a part of these resin will be mellowed by the warmth and will coast out into the tea water. Unmistakably, however, having it boiled in water isn't an effective method to separate oil-solvent materials. The greater part of some recipes include some type of extraction of the cannabis saps into an oil or liquor medium. This is cultivated by any of the accompanying strategies: dousing or boiling in liquor; sautéing or boiling in oil or spread; joining, uncooked, with oil or margarine; mixing, warmed or unheated, with an oil/water emulsion, for example, milk. Milk contains spread fats in emulsion with water. Cannabis materials can be bubbled in milk and will break up into these fats.

Digestion of Cannabis

There are a few different ways an individual can ingest cannabis with shifting degrees of viability. The easiest, however not the most tantalizing, is to bite up and swallow either 5 to 20 grams of cannabis, 1/2 to 2 grams of hashish, or 1/2 gram of hash oil. These sums are dependent upon wide variety due to the tremendously unique potency evaluations of the items accessible and the distinctions in singular resilience.

At the point when these materials are taken straight, you may need to hold up an hour or more, contingent on the action of your digestive system, before the underlying effects are experienced. It requires some less cannabis and time when the material has been appropriately broken down in a reasonable medium. The subsequent point, thusly, is likened to the first. THC is all the more effectively absorbed in the event that it has been broken up in fats or alcohol.

At the point when fats or oils are ingested, the liver gets a sign to emit bile, which is then packed in the gall bladder and launched out into the duodenum. Bile is a viscid, basic liquid which helps in the emulsification, assimilation and ingestion of fats. Cannabis does stimulate the flow of bile, somewhat, If cannabis resins are taken into the body without fat presence, there may not be sufficient bile emitted to achieve their total absorption. In the end, in around two to four fold the number of minutes, some level of the resins will be assimilated.

At the point when food is taken into the stomach it is stirred about while hydrochloric acid and compounds start its processing. After the substance of the stomach become melted, limited quantities of it are shot out into the duodenum at 20-second interims until a specific sum amasses. At that point this procedure of ejection eases back down. Some extremely little amount of fat may now be assimilated straightforwardly into the blood through the intestinal vessels. Next the bile starts its work, emulsifying the fat (scattering it in water in miniscule beads) and rendering a portion of the fatty acid soluble in water. Presently a more prominent measure of these fats can be absorbed through the duodenum. As the processing food is passed from the duodenum to the lower segments of the small digestive tract, a greater amount of the stomach's gastric substance is shot out into the duodenum and likewise followed up on. The all-out procedure of emptying the stomach may take from one to four hours.

Alcohol and Sugar

A solution of alcohol with the cannabis resins is promptly acclimatized even without the digestive system emissions. The stomach serves to a great extent as a food repository in which food is prepared for additional break down. Just a couple of substances, for example, water, alcohol and certain medications, are directly assimilated through this organ. Alcohol is somewhat quickly ingested through the stomach lining and will go about as a vehicle to convey into the body, different substances with which it is combined. Since honey and different sugars are quickly retained into the blood stream through the intestinal vessels, that may likewise serve somewhat as an assimilation vehicle. However, since THC doesn't break down in sugars, the level of ingestion is fairly restricted.

The sign for the stomach to hinder the way toward releasing its substance into the duodenum is brought about by a hormone (enterogastrone). This hormone is discharged from the intestinal mucosa when sugars or potentially fats are available in the small digestive system. If excessive amount of sugar is available, the fats containing the active resins will be kept longer in the stomach.

Choice of Cuisine

The greater part of cannabis ingested will in any case be in the massive wad of food crawling its lazy way through thirty feet of digestive organs. This may have some incentive in that the progressive digestion will assist with keeping up your high for a few hours longer, given that you got enough in you to get stoned on at first. The ingestion pace of your cannabinated food all through its nutritious excursion will be pretty much as follows: 1/3 assimilated during the initial 3 to 4 hours for the underlying high, 1/3 steadily assimilated the following 6 to 8 hours to kind of keep up the high, 1/3 unassimilated materials, which are eventually relinquished to the city sewage framework.

If you need to flush 30 to 40 percent of your overrated grass and hash down the commode, it can be shown by the recipes. In the event that you need to get greater, better, and longer enduring highs for less speculation, at that point read on. From what have been recently examined, a third Guide point can be established: A tad bit of the correct sort of food will help in the assimilation of the cannabis pitches; an excess of food will just weaken its power and waste a lot of it. For a similar explanation that cannabis is best joined with little pieces as opposed to enormous meals, these pieces ought not be taken on a stomach that is now full.

It may be included that the resins of cannabis which are active are rendered increasingly dissolvable (even marginally soluble in water) in a alkaline condition. An acidic condition meddles with their dissolvability. Signs are that the resin is best absorbed, affected by the alkaline juices of the upper piece of the small intestine in the digestive system. In the lower portion of digestive system, absorption is most likely very insignificant. Any further assimilation happening here won't give an extra high, however will just sustain a lazy headache and condition of drowsiness.

Effects of Cooking on Cannabis

The inquiry is now and then posed: "What is the impact of cooking heat upon cannabis? Will it demolish power?" Under typical conditions, there is no considerable loss of strength from cooking. For the most pan, temperatures which would consume or annihilate the active component would as fast ruin the formula itself. Misfortunes of THC strength are normally the aftereffect of oxidation.

Except if cannabis is kept in an airless domain, it will be: subject to oxidation. In a cooler, oxidation rate is nearly invalidated. At room temperature (68°F), oxidation is very progressive. 10% might be lost over a time of a while. At higher temperatures, in the tropics, for example, this deterioration is just marginally higher.

If the cannabis is kept in a hot spot, say 150° or increasingly, a progressively considerable loss of intensity might be normal during a similar measure of time. Cooking temperatures will quicken the oxidizing procedure but, in this case, the lengths of the time typically included are unreasonably short for much misfortune to happen.

In numerous occurrences, it is conceivable that cooking will expand the power of cannabis. In newly harvested hemp, much, and once in a while all, of its THC is available as tetrahydrocannabinol acid. The rate relies on such factors as time of collection and the atmosphere in which it is developed. Unripe cannabis or that developed in northern atmospheres is probably going to contain more THC acid than THC. The acid isn't psychoactive, however after drying quite a bit of it, changes over to THC which is active by a characteristic procedure known as decarboxylation.

The vast majority of the acid remaining will change over to THC during a time of two years. Lamentably, quite a bit of this THC will oxidize in this much time. In the event that the decarboxylation could happen in a condition without oxygen, oxidation would not all the while happen. The utilization of heat can additionally decarboxylate unconverted THC acids in the dried item.

Cannabis and Appetite

A point which ought not be neglected in any treatise on cannabis cooking is the hunger stimulating property of this substance. This has been noted both in clinical examinations and in private use. The smoking of cannabis will regularly give the client a decent instance of the munchies. Yet, when it is ingested, it might just turn such individual into a gastronomical nympho crazy person.

A few cannabises are more disposed to do this than others. So, when you are devouring cannabis, don't leave your pantry be bare. There is much need to likewise call attention to the fact that food can cut you down. In the event that you are too much stoned and need to come down far, a great meal, a not too bad snack or only a tablespoon of honey in warm water will for the most part put your feet closer to the ground. As it has been referenced before, an excessive amount of food in a cannabis dish can crush your high before it even gets an opportunity to occur.

Besides, a few people particularly those with feeble digestive system may get somewhat squeamish when attempting to break down cannabis items. The stomach regularly attempts to eliminate what is hard to process. An excessive amount of food may compound this condition. Regardless of whether you are one of the greater part who has no issue processing cannabinated cooking, an excessive amount of food in the belly can be abominably diverting when you are attempting to encounter euphoria.

CANNABIS AND TASTE

A considerable lot of the antiquated and present-day cannabis preparations are, for the most dish, endeavors at concealing the flavor of cannabis, which numerous persons find unpalatable. Majoun is a commonplace case of this methodology. It is a sugary treat improved and abundantly spiced with cinnamon, cloves, cardamom, nutmeg or different ingredients which satisfactorily, if not completely, mask the hemp flavor.

A portion of these recipes have been included in light of the fact that they are heavenly and trustworthy, also classical. The vast majority of some recipes, in any case, are concocted upon the reason that the kind of cannabis is tasty when prepared accurately and joined with different ingredients which are agreeable with its essence. A significant number of these recipes treat cannabis as a topping without which the flavor of the preparation would certainly endure.

CHAPTER THREE: HEALTHY AND IMPROVED LIVING WITH CANNABIS DIET/ FOODS

For quite a long time, there have deception about a plant that is nothing short of life-saving in several cases. You should be open to the possibility that cannabis is something other than a weed with an undeserved notoriety — it's a plant that really holds the ability to improve your life.

IMPROVING SLEEP

In any event, when we believe we're getting enough rest, ecological components like light, sound, and stress can influence the nature of that rest, decreasing the estimation of the hours we spend in bed and conceivably leaving us feeling groggier than previously. Some few things are more disappointing than making an opportunity to hit the sheets early just to wind up lying conscious, considering the condition of the world until three toward the beginning of the day. Or then again you may nod off rapidly however, you find yourself waking up irregularly, maybe in view of a wheezing partner or annoying pain. Whatever is shielding you from getting a decent night's rest, interfered with rest can be significantly tiring and can leave you feeling weak and exhausted.

Encountering an unpleasant night's rest from time to time is normal. However, a few people are troubled by sleep disorders that can unleash ruin on everyday lives. Insomnia, rest apnea, restless leg condition, and narcolepsy are only a couple of regular disorders of sleep that can be brought about by a mix of components which range from physical and clinical issues to mental disorders and environmental variables. They additionally accompany severe reactions that can include uneasiness, depression, exhaustion, low immunity, hormonal disturbance, and hallucinations. While pharmaceuticals can offer alleviation for a portion of these conditions, they frequently accompany their own problematic side effects.

Having poor sleep can possibly crash a sound way of life, so revising a flawed rest plan is the most ideal approach to improve wellbeing and health. Many doctors have clarified that one of the primary side effects they hope to treat, paying little heed to the condition or disorder being referred to, is their patients' weariness and exhaustion. It is shown that it is the most significant course in reestablishing their patients to ideal degrees of wellbeing, since whenever the body has the chance to rest appropriately, it can recuperate all the more viably and all the more productively.

How Cannabis Can Help

While there's no contending with the way that cannabis influences rest, scientists are as yet attempting to figure out which phases of sleep are influenced by cannabis, and which mix of compounds of the plant are well on the way to assist somebody with accomplishing a long, fulfilling night of sleep. These are cannabinoids, the powerful component in cannabis that give it its therapeutic worth. The most ordinarily explored cannabinoids are THC (tetrahydrocannabinol) and CBD (cannabidiol), and both have been appeared to have applications as tranquilizers.

There are a couple of things we can say without a doubt about cannabis and sleep. One of cannabis' most well-known cannabinoids, THC, has been appeared to drastically build melatonin creation in the brain, a hormone occurring naturally that controls the body's circadian rhythm. When cannabinoids like THC and CBD enter the body, they impersonate compounds made by the body, called endocannabinoids. These neurochemicals are a basic part of the body's endocannabinoid framework, which is answerable for a large group of substantial capacities, including the guideline of rest.

DECREASING STRESS AND ANXIETY

Nowadays, it's anything but difficult to direct our repressed feelings of stress and tension to long days at the workplace, bothering issues in our own personal relationships or monetary burdens like vehicle repair or credit card bills. Stress is readily seen in a negative light: Individuals may put to blame their tension for failure to function optimally at work, or worry for trouble in sinking into serene reflection.

Stress to portray a physical strain on the human body. Stress can affect one's wellbeing. The body reacts to stress in three phases: alarm, resistance, and weariness. Anxiety, however firmly related, isn't a similar thing as stress. While stress is the body's reaction to a current stressor and can bring about horde sentiments like annoyance, trouble, or worry, anxiety happens without a stressor and is related essentially with fear and apprehensions. Once in a while it's anything but difficult to distinguish the reasons for anxiety; different occasions, it comes flying out of fantasy land.

In spite of the fact that the vast majority experience anxiety in waves, being in a condition of ceaseless anxiety resembles leaving your fight-or-flight reaction turned on inconclusively. If not tended to, that drawn out impact can add to the improvement of anxiety disorders that can make continuing with typical life appear to be close to unthinkable. Summed up anxiety disorder, social anxiety disorder, panic disorder, obsessive-compulsive disorder, PTSD, and explicit fears all fit under the anxiety umbrella. Anyway, you characterize them, stress and anxiety are a critical, and rising issue.

How Cannabis Can Help

Specialists are attempting to sort out how cannabis functions in the body to mitigate anxiety. The subsequent examinations to date have shown that cannabis and its most regularly researched compounds, the cannabinoids THC and CBD, can adjust anxiety on a portion subordinate premise.

The endocannabinoid framework, or ECS, is a significant regulatory system that exists in each warm-blooded animal. It starts both mental and physiological changes as our bodies adjust to new situations or conditions—consider stress simply one more situation that our bodies are continually attempting to adjust to. Stress and anxiety will actuate a healthy ECS with the goal that it produces endocannabinoids—that is, the cannabinoids in our bodies—varying. These endocannabinoids then initiate the endocannabinoid receptors found all through our bodies to encourage the important reaction.

An uneven ECS can cause issues, particularly with regards to psychological wellness. In 2014, analysts at Vanderbilt University had the option to affirm that when individuals endured incessant pressure or serious emotional injury, they were in danger of a decrease in their endocannabinoid production, which in this way expanded their odds of encountering anxiety. This is the place the cannabinoids from cannabis can prove to be useful.

A similar report found that when clients who were inadequate in endocannabinoids ingest cannabis, their anxiety was diminished. THC and CBD act along these lines to the body's endocannabinoids, which means they can open or fit into cannabinoid receptors similarly. At a neurochemical level, taking in cannabinoids like THC and CBD can assist with directing the body's ECS by attempting to reestablish balance. As we referenced before, however, the dose level has a huge influence: an excessive amount of cannabis, it turns out, upsets the ECS and can expand anxiety.

Finding the line among expanding and diminishing one's anxiety with the use of cannabis has a ton to do with the qualities of the plant's predominant compounds. It is known that THC is the cannabinoid liable for the euphoric feeling or high, that accompanies ingesting cannabis, and for some first-time clients, this inclination isn't generally lovely—actually, some reprimand it for causing them to feel progressively on edge. CBD, in a way, doesn't cause euphoria. This reality alone has some persuaded that CBD may be more successful than THC at treating anxiety.

METABOLISM, WEIGHT MANAGEMENT, AND EXERCISE RECOVERY

The undeniably regular use and underwriting of cannabis by competitors, wellness lovers, and health specialists is crushing the badly educated idea that over the top cannabis use prompts ridiculous craving, laziness, and weight gain. In any case, before comprehension can be held on what new research says about the connection among cannabis and your waistline, how about the need to highlight the three zones that researchers concur have colossal potential with regards to restorative cannabis use.

Metabolism is basically the procedure answerable for changing over the nutrients in what was eaten, into the energy required to do work. At the point when energy isn't required, it's put away in the body for some other time. An individual's metabolic rate relies upon various components, including yet not restricted to muscle mass, tallness and weight, age, hereditary qualities, exercise propensities, and diet. While metabolism is a progressing physiological procedure, weight management is tied in with attempting to remain inside a healthy range, in a perfect world by keeping up a sound eating regimen and level of physical activity.

If you work out, you'll realize that an exercise can prompt sore muscles that leave you feeling not exactly roused to get up the following day and repeat a similar daily practice. Athletes at professional levels who don't have the alternative of resting through a morning routine depend on various stunts and methods to accelerate their athletic recuperation, helping them get back in the game all the more rapidly.

How Cannabis Can Help

As outlandish as it might appear to a few, the most recent research on the connection between cannabis use and metabolism shows a couple of things. In the first place, the plant has far more noteworthy potential as an enhancement for weight regulation than recently suspected conceivable; and second, in the more extensive sense, regardless of whether one knows about the side effects or not, casual cannabis use after some time can prompt a progressively stable body weight and even a littler waistline. The examination on the connection between cannabis use and metabolism implies that, in spite of cannabis clients' conceivably ingesting a larger number of calories than nonusers, it doesn't appear to influence their wellbeing in an antagonistic manner.

AN EFFECTIVE SOURCE OF PAIN MANAGEMENT

Being in a prolonged condition of physical pain isn't entertaining. Beside producing a terrible inclination in the body, pain additionally influences our psychological state, and how one sees things. Interminable pain is regularly neuropathic, which means it is brought about by harm to or infection of the body's somatosensory sensory system (the piece of the sensory system that detects your environment), yet it can likewise be nociceptive, or brought about by harm to tissue. While patients portray the former as a shooting or intense pain, the latter will in general feel increasingly like arching or pulsating, and is regularly part of the body's irritation reaction to contamination, wounds, or tissue harm.

For momentary pain, it's basic for us to incline toward over-the-counter prescriptions like acetaminophen (Tylenol) or ibuprofen (Advil) to help diminish the pain. While these medications absolutely have their place in treating pain, abuse can prompt harmful hepatitis, ulcers, interior dying, and other unfavorable effects. Progressively serious nociceptive pain may be treated with a narcotic, a similarly significant sort of medication in our pharmacopeia, however one that, when overprescribed and unmanaged, can have critical results. Pharmaceutical medications have unquestionably become the standard of care, and keeping in mind that it may appear as if cannabis is simply rising as a characteristic pain reliever, truly it's been utilized to help oversee pain for in excess of 5,000 years.

How Cannabis Can Help

The topic of whether cannabis can be a valuable device for the management pain isn't begging to be proven wrong: a huge number of long periods of its utilization as a pain relieving joined with many patient self-report reviews produced in the course of the most recent years reveal to us that individuals who use cannabis experience help from pain, regardless of whether neuropathic or nociceptive.

While historical use has directed us toward cannabis for relief from discomfort, researchers are as yet attempting to see correctly how cannabis functions in this unique circumstance with the goal that it very well may be utilized successfully. Fortunately, a more noteworthy acknowledgment of the plant as a pain reliever lately has prompted better quality research regarding the matter of precisely what cannabis, and all the more explicitly cannabinoids, do in the body to help control pain.

In a 2017 clinical survey distributed in the journal, Cannabis and Cannabinoid Research, it was affirmed that different randomized, controlled clinical preliminaries show that cannabis can be a viable pharmacotherapy for pain. The literature demonstrated that, when contrasted with a placebo treatment, cannabinoids were related with a more prominent decrease in torment and more noteworthy normal decrease in numerical pain evaluations.

The body's endocannabinoid framework assumes a significant job in the administration of pain and inflammation While the body's regular endocannabinoids are created on an on-request premise in harmed tissues to help decrease pain by enacting our cannabinoid receptors, cannabinoids like THC and CBD can similarly affect our pain resistance.

THC is an incomplete agonist of both CB1 and CB2 receptors, which means it goes about as an "activator," starting a physical reaction. It is explained that neurotic pain states have been proposed to emerge, at any rate to some degree, from a dysregulation of the endocannabinoid system, implying that an uneven ECS may be at any rate mostly at fault for progressing pain.

This is inferred that fundamental science and clinical preliminaries bolster the possibility that cannabinoid treatment is a functional method to treat constant pain. While we realize that cannabinoids like THC and CBD can assist us with managing various kinds of pain, researchers have (generally) reasoned that what makes cannabinoids viable isn't really how they communicate with the pain itself, however how they interface with our impression of the pain we're encountering.

A POWERFUL SUPPORT FOR CANCER TREATMENT

Despite the fact that regularly alluded to as a solitary malady, there are in excess of a hundred kinds of cancer. But from leukemia to melanoma, and breast malignancy to prostate disease, they all start similarly. Malignant growth begins at a cell level, when cells in the tissues of our body start to act unusually, developing, working, and separating—yet not kicking the bucket, similar to typical cells should.

A development of these irregular cells can shape a tumor; however, tumors are not a trait of each sort of cancer. Tumors that are not dangerous are named benign, and once they've been evacuated, it's improbable that they'll return. A malignant tumor, may however, return in light of the fact that carcinogenic cells can go through different pieces of the body — like, through the circulatory system—and spread to different regions. This is the reason early discovery of disease is so significant.

The physical impacts of cancer can shift starting with one individual then onto the next, regardless of whether two individuals have a similar sort of disease. Weariness, pain, sickness, change in appetite, rest issues, and an absence of enthusiasm for sex are largely basic reactions, yet not every person with cancer growth will encounter them.

Life-saving medications like chemotherapy and radiation are genuinely requesting and can fuel these side effects exponentially.

The joined impact of cancer and its treatment on the body is surely crippling, however the impact of a malignancy finding on the psyche is similarly harming. A diagnosis of cancer essentially expands an individual's risk of creating anxiety and depression and frequently leaves patients with a sentiment of sadness and sorrow that appears to be unconquerable.

Normal cancer treatment incorporates chemotherapy, which utilizes a progression of medications to execute disease cells, and radiation, which utilizes high-energy waves like X-beams, gamma beams, or charged particles to wreck or harm malignant growth cells. While these standard medicines and treatments are unquestionably compelling, they likewise harm solid cells in the body, and, as expressed prior, can add to and intensify the reactions of the cancer.

Directed treatment is another treatment that is utilized to obstruct the activity of specific compounds, proteins, or particles that are engaged with the spread of malignant growth, while hormone treatment includes, squares, or expels hormones to help prevent disease cells from proceeding to replicate, or to slow their generation. Treatment is absolutely not restricted to these four techniques, however, with patients frequently enhancing them with reciprocal and elective meds to help improve their personal satisfaction.

How Cannabis Can Help

Talking about the connection among cannabis and cancer takes a touch of artfulness. While cannabis has been viewed as an advantageous type of treatment for cancer and its manifestations for quite a few years, droves of supposed cannabis experts have spread some genuine deception about cannabis and cancer. More regrettable, this information isn't just false, it additionally can possibly cause added damage to patients who are likely previously enduring with the impacts of a terminal sickness.

At the point when enacted, the endocannabinoid receptors situated all through the body (both CB1 and CB2) decimate cells by initiating something many refer to as apoptosis, or "cell self-destruction." "This happens inside the body while shielding the healthy cells from the harming impacts of chemotherapy and radiation. This is appeared in a recent report distributed in the Journal of Exploratory Research in Pharmacology, which noticed that while cannabis has been utilized in the palliative treatment of cancer for quite a while, headways in research on the endocannabinoid system have indicated that cannabinoids can be powerful enemy of tumor agents in view of their capacity to instigate apoptosis, what's more, advance cell development hindrance.

A few studies have discovered that cannabinoids incite apoptosis in both in vitro models (in a petri dish) and in vivo (in living beings), and records a few distributions that report effectively treating forceful tumors along these lines.

One thing that makes cannabinoid treatment for cancer appealing to doctors and oncologists is that it can secure healthy cells in the body while easing back tumor development and killing disease cells. Also, that is not all. Starter information shows that cannabis can synergistically affect conventional cancer treatment like chemotherapy and radiation, making them work all the more adequately.

EASING THE AGING PROCESS

As much as individuals know maturing is unavoidable, many people will do pretty much anything to attempt to leave it speechless—from typical things like applying sunscreen and eating well to progressively exceptional undertakings like getting placenta facials or having blood infusions. Obviously, aging goes a long way past the physical—and to be honest, one is progressively keen on what he/she can do to shield oneself from Alzheimer's infection, stroke, or knee replacement than a couple of chuckle lines or crow's feet. From joint pain to dementia to Parkinson's malady, the rundown of ailments related with aging is long, and the side effects of such sicknesses can affect an individual's personal satisfaction, particularly they're being influenced by more than each disease in turn, which is frequently the situation.

How Cannabis Can Help

Pain and cancer are two regions that make up an impressive number of conditions influencing seniors, and are a piece of the motivation behind why cannabis is picking up such a great amount of notoriety among this gathering — cannabis can give alleviation from numerous infirmities without a moment's delay! Notwithstanding, encountering constant pain or cancer, an individual moving toward end of life may feel anxious, fear or depression and cannabis can do some incredible things with regards to placing those emotions into point of view.

Truth be told, caregivers regularly report that end of-life cannabis use enables old patients to accommodate with the way that they're going to bite the dust. Furthermore, if one recall the significance of sleep and the manner in which a decent night's rest can in numerous cases be improved with a little cannabis, we can perceive how a few points previously secured can loan themselves to use of cannabis among seniors.

Not many investigations have indicated that cannabis may assist with overseeing behavioral side effects related with these conditions. A published review in the diary Current Neurology and Neuroscience Reports found that in past writing, while manufactured THC end up being similarly as powerful as different drugs utilized for dementia, a few contextual investigations found that it was a predominant medication.

It is said that given different advantages related with cannabis use, it was a superior treatment for behavioral issues related with dementia than ordinary prescriptions like antipsychotics, which have been appeared to expand the risk of mortality because of cardiovascular occasions just as desire (unintentionally taking in remote issue).

CHAPTER FOUR: PREPARATIONS OF MATERIALS FOR CANNABIS AND ITS RECIPES

Cannabis items are gotten from the female Cannabis sativa or C. Indica plant. The psychoactive substance in cannabis is called tetrahydrocannabinol (THC). In India and other Eastern countries cannabis items come in four fundamental forms: ganjah (the resin secured bloom tops), bhang (the leaves from underneath the tops), chars (the resin assembled from the tops), and hashish or mimea (the tars removed with fat in boiling water and solidified). A portion of these names mean various things in various areas. The terms bhang and hashish, in certain spots, are given to inebriating refreshments rnade from cannabis.

In the United States and most Western countries the accessible cannabis items are marijuana, hashish and hash oil. The term cannabis alludes to every usable piece of the plant. The entire flower tops with zero broken leafy material is normally the strongest and costly type of this item. This wrecked verdant material might be either shakes (the strong crumblings from the dry tops) or the less intense leaves from the lower portions of the plant. An ordinary example of better than average quality cannabis sold on the American black market would comprise of roughly equivalent parts of tops and shakes with a generous measure of seeds included.

Hashish as a term here includes both the fat removed hashish or mimea and the assembled resins. The expression "charas" is once in a while utilized in America. Now and then this item is wrongly called "kif or pollen hash". Kif is really a mix of ganjah and dark tobacco prepared in Morocco. Pollen, obviously, originates from the male, as opposed to the female, plant. Hashish might be 5 to multiple times as powerful as the cannabis from which it was determined. Hash oil is a dissolvable extraction of the active oils and saps from either hashish or cannabis. There are various evaluations of hash oil controlled by the level of refinement and the level of active THC.

Earthy colored oil is the crudest extraction; however, it might be 2 to multiple times as concentrated as the hashish from which it came. Refinements of higher nature includes red oil, golden oil, honey oil, and white oil, in a specific order. A cutting-edge procedure known as isomerization may additionally build the intensity of hash oil without diminishing its volume.

This procedure convenes one of the inert components of the oil to active THC and simultaneously changes the lower pivoting THC particle to a higher turning and progressively potent isomer. These transformations may expand the intensity by as much as multiple times and furthermore improve the nature of the high. Isomerization evacuates a significant part of the overwhelming qualities which are sleep inducing from cannabis and permits an increasingly light and elevating high.

BASIC MATERIAL FOR CANNABIS RECIPES

These materials are helpful in the preparation of quick acting and powerful cannabis recipes. It isn't completely vital, however, that these materials be close by. In the event that you appreciate smoking cannabis and have not too bad cooking skills, you have nothing to stress over with regards to cannabis food aside from choosing what to make first. Then again, you love cannabis but need a formula to have water boiled, at that point never fear, on the grounds that in this area you will be presented with the extremely essential strategies you should learn so as to begin and get stoned without any long time of study.

What's more, if you truly stall out, recall, it's much simpler to get high with a little assistance from your companions, especially the ones who realize how to boil water by heart. In any case, since cannabis is most effortlessly infused into staples through oil or margarine, the basic recipes required to play out this hallucinogenic imbuement are actually all you have to know. Cannabis spread (cannabutter) can be utilized in any cooking that calls for margarine, with results that lift even the most unassuming food to a holy observance of the most high. Obviously, you can likewise simply spread some cannabutter on a cut of toast, however, that doesn't really sound fun at all.

On the whole, some basic standards. Discover a strategy for infusion that works for you and make use of it, utilizing a supply of cannabutter which is consistent, cannacoconut oil, or THC oil to make the appetizers, meals, and treats depicted in this book however much as could reasonably be expected. You certainly don't need any shocks with regards to the power of your product.

THC OIL (CANNABIS-INFUSED OIL)

It's not important to utilize first-squeezed extra-virgin or bequest packaged olive oil to make your THC Oil; a reasonable virgin olive oil works pleasantly. Obviously, top notch ingredients bring about an increasingly flavorful finished result, so if you plan on utilizing your THC Oil for serving of mixed greens dressings or to sprinkle over veggies and pasta, a fruity extra-virgin olive oil will have a significant effect.

Ingredients: Makes 6 cups. 6 cups olive oil or canola oil, 1-ounce cannabis buds, finely ground, or 2 ounces cut leaf, dried and ground.

Instructions:

In a twofold evaporator, gradually heat oil on low warmth for a couple of moments until you start to smell the oil's fragrance. Include the ground cannabis gradually, mixing until it is completely covered before including more cannabis. Stew on low heat for 45 minutes, mixing every so often. Have the blend removed from heat and permit it to cool before straining. Press the plant matter with the rear of a spoon to wring all the oil out of it. Compost the verdant remains and have the oil kept in an impermeable holder in the fridge for as long as 2 months.

CANNACOCONUT OIL

Coconut oil has a ton of preferences over animal products. It's a saturated fat, permitting most extreme ingestion of cannabinoids, however it's substantially more empowering for you than animal fat that is saturated. Coconut oil is certainly the best alternative for vegetarians and those worried about health. Accessible at health food stores and all around loaded markets, it's strong at room temperature however liquefies without any problem.

Ingredients: Makes 1¾ cups. 1 ounce cannabis, dried, or 2 ounces cut leaf, One 14-ounce container coconut oil.

Instructions:

Fill a huge stockpot with water, and include your cannabis. Make it simmer over low heat, mixing sometimes, for 60 minutes. At that point, include your coconut oil, and come back to simmer. Place away from heat. Let the coconut oil blend, sit for two days as it gradually extracts, in a secured pot at room temperature. At that point, warm the oil, cannabis, and water blend until the oil liquefies. Strain the blend, being certain to press the plant matter immovably against the side of the sifter.

Refrigerate the oil and water blend for at any rate 24 hours. Return the following day and separate the hardened oil from the water. Pat dry with a paper towel, at that point dissolve the cannacoconut oil in a pan until it is fluid. Measure into glass containers for simple dosing. You can make use of baby food jars.

CANNABIS-INFUSED MAYONNAISE

This sauce already emulsified, requires around ten minutes of constant whisking to appropriately blend the ingredients, so be patient and include the oil gradually, actually drop by drop, in case the sauce "break" and neglect to emulsify. You can likewise utilize a food processor, including the oil drop by drop through the feeder tube while the processor is running; in any case, the texture of the mayo is normally lighter when the whisking is done by hand.

Make it certain to give this recipe a run through once without the cannabis, in order to get the feel for legitimate oil-yolk emulsification, in such a case that the mayo "breaks" with the ganja in it—well, that could be a money related chomp. Additionally, since the eggs are not cooked in this recipe, make it certain to get natural, local, ranch new eggs, and if such eggs are inaccessible, utilize pasteurized eggs to keep away from any danger of salmonella. You should make use of pasteurized eggs or keep away from custom made mayo if your immune system is easily compromised.

Ingredients: 1 cup soybean oil, ½ ounce ganja shake, 2 enormous egg yolks, 1 teaspoon new lemon juice, Pinch of salt, 1 teaspoon white vinegar, ½ teaspoon Dijon mustard

Instructions:

In a twofold heater, mix the oil and cannabis. Heat over low until the cannabis smell is strong yet not burnt or nutty. The oil ought to have a gritty green tint to it. Let cool. Remove and have the herb strained, crushing the weed in a metal sifter against the work with the rear of a spoon to wring out each drop of oil. Ensure that every one of your ingredients have been brought to room temperature—this is significant!

In a little metal bowl, make use of an immersion blender or rush to altogether mix the egg yolks, lemon juice, salt, vinegar, and mustard (this should likewise be possible in a food processor or blender). Utilizing a ½ teaspoon measure, gradually include the implanted oil, a couple of drops one after another, while continually mixing on low or whisking until the mayo is thick and beginning to shape strips.

If it's excessively thick, you can include room-temperature water in little augmentation. If your blend "breaks," it tends to be fixed by whisking some more space temperature egg yolks in a different bowl, at that point gradually whisking those yolks into the "broken" mayo blend. If that still doesn't work, include a couple of drops of high temperature water. Have it covered and chill; keep in the fridge for 4 to 5 days.

SIMPLE CANNABUTTER

This is a simple, speedy approach to mix cannabis into butter on your burner. Be certain to utilize salted butter since it has a higher smoke point, and be careful not to leave your pot unattended! You can make this cannabutter rapidly, and use it in any recipe of your choice.

Ingredients: Makes ½ cup. ½ cup (1 stick) salted butter, ¼ ounce cannabis buds, finely ground. To make cannamargarine, essentially substitute margarine for butter in this recipe.

Instructions:

The butter should be melted on low heat in a pan. Include the ground buds, and on a low heat medium, simmer for 45 minutes, mixing frequently. The butter should then be strained into a glass dish with a tight-fitting cover. Push the rear of a spoon against the plant matter, and crush it against the sifter to press out each drop of butter you can get. At the point when you're set, dispose of the plant matter. Utilize your cannabutter quickly, or refrigerate or freeze until the time has come to make use of it. You can undoubtedly scale this recipe up for bigger groups of cannabutter. 1 pound of margarine (4 sticks) can ingest 1 ounce of cannabis, yet you might need to simmer for as long as an hour. Shower this cannabutter over newly cooked pasta or popcorn for instant fulfillment. Hold enormous clusters in the cooler for use in recipes.

CANNABUTTER FROM SEEDS

The external part of cannabis seed structures is genuinely rich in THC. Within the seed contains just protein. dampness, and the nonactive fixed oil. The seeds are very nutritious and have been utilized by man for food in certain parts of the world. The best thing that should be possible with seeds that are good, obviously, is to plant them. This for different reasons, isn't generally practicable.

Cannabutter can be set up by simmering 1 cup of seeds in 1/2 pound of margarine at a low temperature for around 5 minutes. Due to their nonporous texture, it is simpler to strain the butter from the seeds than from the leaves. Likewise, there are not really any basic oils or terpenes on the seeds. The resultant cannnabutter is basically tasteless and can be utilized either by people who don't support the flavor of cannabis.

WAMM CANNABIS FLOUR

The Wo/Men's Alliance for Medical Marijuana is a progressive clinical cannabis aggregate that endeavors to satisfy the humane objectives of California's pivotal Proposition 215 voter activity, which previously legitimized clinical cannabis in the state in 1996. At WAMM, patients with terminal and interminable ailments volunteer to help tend an enormous outdoor natural cannabis garden, which they collect and then process into their own medication.

All aspects of the plant are utilized, including the stems that go into tincture, the leaves ground into flour for heating, and even a couple of seeds for planting the following year's nursery. It isn't encouraging to strain the entire plant fiber away from the oil or margarine. Rather, the cannabis leaves are pummeled totally that the subsequent product is a superfine filtered flour that breaks down directly into butter and oil. Utilizing the entire plant along these lines gives additional fiber and nutrients.

Ingredients: Makes around 25 grams. 1 ounce leaf material (least)

Equipment: Latex gloves, 145-micron silk screen mounted on a wooden casing, bit of glass or mirror bigger than silk screen

Instructions:

To crush the cannabis flour, first of all, get your plants harvested, regardless of whether they are indoor or outside. Trim the leaves and dry them topsy turvy or on a screen, in a warm, dry, dim spot for a week or somewhere in the vicinity, until they are totally dry. At that point, utilize a blender to crush the leaves into powder, cautiously mixing with a metal spread knife kept well over the blender's blades. A vortex will shape in the blender, and you should cautiously mix more cannabis from the sides of the blender into this vortex.

It takes around 5 minutes to get the cannabis finely ground. Turn off the blender each 1 or 2 minutes so it doesn't overheat, and with the knife, stir up the blended, ground cannabis. Next, the product is poured over a fine silk screen extended on a wooden edge. Beneath the screen, there ought to be a glass or mirror. Utilize your gloved hands or a plastic card to rub the ground leaf over the screen. Evacuate any stems quickly, as they can cut the screen and make an opening. Keep scouring the leaf over the screen until, in any event, 50 percent of the leaf has gone through.

Presently, gather all the leaf that despite everything hasn't been screened and returned it in the blender. Mix again for 5 minutes, until the leaf is ground more finely. Pour this twice-mixed item over the screen once more, and resume scouring it through. When you have around 30 percent of that clump staying, gather it from the highest point of the screen and mix once more. When the leaf has been mixed multiple times, it is as fine as anyone might imagine.

Rub it over the screen once more, and any outstanding pieces too enormous to fit through the screen ought to be evacuated and put aside for making tinctures. Make use of a card to scratch all the ground flour off the screen into an enormous plastic water/air proof compartment. Remove the screen and uncover the ultrafine finished cannabis flour underneath. Cautiously scratch the flour off the glass with a card, and store in an impenetrable plastic or glass compartment.

Tinctures

At their simplest form, tinctures are just plant matter immersed in alcohol . Your nearby health food store has numerous tinctures of various restorative plants accessible, such as damiana and echinacea. Tinctures are a phenomenal method to ingest cannabis for a couple of key reasons: They are entirely convenient and cautious, you maintain a tend to do away with additional calories from therapeutic pastries or greasy THC-oil-doused meals, and it's anything but difficult to gauge your portion. Just press the dropper top, and discharge the dropper underneath your tongue.

Let it stay there for a few minutes. This is the place it's least demanding for the tincture to be absorbed. You'll start feeling the effect in around ten to thirty minutes, so tinctures are quicker acting than having to digest a medible. Basic tinctures made with vodka or rum can turn into the base for cannabis mixed drinks. Tinctures can be made by utilizing any cannabis item, from stems to the best kif. The suggested soaking times are typically long, as long as two months in some cannabis tincture.

It will take more time to ingest all the THC from woody plant parts like stems than from finely filtered ground bud or kif. Another issue to consider is whether to utilize alcohol or glycerin. Alcohol appears to make an increasingly powerful tincture, however it burns under the tongue and tastes like medication in old times. Glycerin tastes sweet and unlike alcohol, doesn't burn, so it very well may be simpler to utilize.

QUICK CANNABIS GLYCERITE

This is a quicker form of a glycerin-based cannabis tincture. A few cooks accept that you should heat the blend for greatest potency, and that essentially soaking your herb in glycerin isn't sufficient.

Ingredients: Makes 1 cup. ¼ ounce top notch cannabis shake, ½ cup in addition to 1 tablespoon USP food-grade glycerin, 6 tablespoons water

Equipment: Latex gloves, unbleached cheesecloth, big glass container with tight cover

Instructions:

All ingredients should be combined in a Crockpot, and simmer at an exceptionally low temperature (about 180°F) for 2½ hours. Place away from heat and permit to cool until it tends to be handled securely. With latex gloves on, strain, and at that point press the cannabis glycerite well through unbleached cheesecloth into an enormous glass container with a tight cover. Store in a cool, dull spot for as long as a half year.

Equipment for Preparation

For the recipes which are basic, you'll need a saucepan or that for frying. Stay away from aluminum and Teflon coated cookware at whatever point conceivable for cast iron or hardened steel. A double boiler is additionally useful, and if you don't have one helpful, it's extremely simply a question of discovering one pot that will settle inside another, with the goal that you can boil water in the lower level as an approach to exactly and uniformly heat the margarine or oil in the upper level. Likewise, look for a glass or Pyrex estimating cup and a metal fine-mesh strainer. Try not to utilize a plastic sifter, as hot oil may soften it.

At last, it's useful to have a coffee processor or blender committed to separating your cannabis, however scissors or a hand processor will get the job done. Furthermore, you'll additionally need an exact scale for measuring and estimating your important hash, buds, or leaves. Crock-pots are extremely valuable when making enormous clumps of cannabutter, just as for other recipes and can be found nationwide.

Blenders, food processors, juicers, and frozen yogurt producers are additionally fun kitchen toys that can be gotten easily in market. Other important items are kitchen utensils you'll require include measuring spoons, spatula, scoop, wooden spoons, blending bowls, heating container, cheesecloth, and a meat thermometer for preparing food securely. A candy thermometer is basic for making caramels and hard It.

CHAPTER FIVE: CANNABIS RECIPES

Cannabis Buttercream Frosting

Ingredients: Makes enough icing to cover two 9-inch round cakes. ½ cup unsalted Simple Cannabutter, 1 pound confectioners' sugar (about 3 cups), 4 to 5 tablespoons substantial cream or milk, 1 teaspoon vanilla concentrate.

Instructions:

The cannabutter is first brought to room temperature until it is strong however, not hard. When it has arrived at the correct consistency, gradually mix it in an enormous bowl with the confectioners' sugar, 4 tablespoons cream, and vanilla. Utilizing an electric blender is most straightforward but, the mixing should be possible by hand. Beat until smooth, including more cream until the icing appears to be anything but difficult to spread. This frosting is quite useful and can be utilized on a cooled cake.

Jack Herer Hemp Cookies

A recipe from Mary Aught-Six, Author of The Emperor Wears No Clothes, an earth-shattering book about hemp that started a grassroots development, Jack Herer was a resolute champion of the cannabis plant. Herer utilized cannabis as a medication and as motivation while venturing to the far corners of the planet prompting individuals to relegalize the hemp plant so they could profit by its bunch of modern uses, including for food, biofuel, construction and textile materials, and also body-care items.

Ingredients:

Makes 24 cookiess. 1½ cups (3 sticks) canna margarine, 2¼ cups hemp flour, 1½ teaspoons baking soda, 1 teaspoon sea salt, ¼ cup packed light brown colored sugar, 2 cups Splenda granulated sugar or proportional normal sugar substitution, 1½ teaspoons vanilla concentrate, 3 eggs, 3 cups five-grain rolled oat, 1 cup walnut halves, coarsely sliced, 1 cup dried cranberries, 1 cup broiled hemp seed, 1 cup golden raisins.

Instructions:

In a double boiler, liquefy cannamargarine over medium heat. Keeping warming over low heat for 45 minutes to 60 minutes, until the cannabis is earthy colored and fresh. Preheat the stove to 375°F. Daintily oil two cookie sheets and put in a safe spot. In an enormous bowl, filter together hemp flour, baking soda, and salt.

In another bowl, mix the liquefied cannamargarine, earthy colored sugar, sweetener, vanilla, and ¾ cup water together. Beat eggs and add to cannamargarine blend, at that point mix into the flour blend. Include grain, walnuts, dried cranberries, hemp seed, and raisins. Blend well.

Place your batter into pecan size pieces and arrange on the baking sheets. Heat for 10 to 12 minutes. Cookies ought to be delicate in the middle, with light earthy colored edges. Cool on racks.

Budder Cookies Recipe

Ingredients: 3 cups flour, 1-pound canna margarine, soft, 1 cup sugar, powdered 1 tbsp. vanilla, 1/4 c. granulated sugar

Instructions:

At first, combine margarine with sugar and vanilla, include flour bit by bit. Distribute onto cookie sheet secured with material paper. Press delicately with a ramekin then sprinkle with granulated sugar. Cook at 125 C for 10 minutes. Set aside to cool totally.

Canna-Oatmeal Raisin Cookies

Ingredients:

24 1/4 cup cannabis margarine, ¾ cup normal butter, 1 cup brown sugar, 1 cup white sugar, 2 eggs, 1 teaspoon vanilla concentrate, 2 cups brisk cooking oats, 2 cups universally handy flour, 1 teaspoon baking soda, 1 teaspoon heating powder, 1 teaspoon salt, 1 cup raisins, 1 cup dried cranberries.

Instructions:

Beat cannabis butter and that of the normal, sugars, eggs and vanilla for 5 minutes. Using another bowl, join oats, flour, baking soda and powder, salt. Add to the earlier mixture of butter, and 1 cup at once. Blend in raisins and cranberries. Drop by spoonful onto lubed cookie sheets and prepare for 12-14 minutes at 350 degrees F.

Vegan Cannabis Carrot Muffins

Ingredients:

Makes 24 muffins. ½ cup liquefied coconut oil, 24 grams cannabis shake, 1¾ cups generally useful flour, ½ teaspoon salt, ¼ teaspoon baking soda, ⅛ teaspoon baking powder, 1 teaspoon ground cinnamon, ½ teaspoon ground nutmeg, 1 teaspoon ground ginger, 1 tablespoon new lemon juice, ½ cup soy milk, 1 cup maple syrup, 1 teaspoon vanilla concentrate 2 cups finely slashed carrots, ½ cup squashed pineapple, well drained, ½ cup golden raisins, ½, cup sliced coconut, ½ cup finely diced walnuts.

Instructions:

Preheat the broiler to 350°F. Line muffins tins with 3-ounce heating cups. Put in a safe spot. Coconut oil is combined and shake in a pan. Simmer over low heat for 30 minutes. Strain through a metal sifter, squeezing the cannabis against the sides to remove all the oil, and cool. In a blending bowl, filter together flour, salt, baking soda and powder, cinnamon, nutmeg, and ginger.

In a different bowl, whisk together lemon juice, soy milk, maple syrup, and vanilla. Empty wet ingredients into the dry ones. Whisk until blended. Overlap in carrots, pineapple, raisins, coconut, and walnuts.

Spoon batter into prepared muffin tins. Prepare 20 to 25 minutes or until a toothpick embedded into the center of muffin comes out and the muffins are colored golden on top. Cool totally.

Classic Cannabis Brownies

Ingredients:

1 cup all-purpose flour, ¼ cup unsweetened cocoa powder, ½ teaspoon baking powder, ¼ teaspoon salt, 3 tablespoons THC Oil, 5 ounce semisweet chocolate, cleaved 1½ tablespoons light corn syrup, 1 cup packed brown sugar, 1 tablespoon fruit pure, 3 egg whites, 2 teaspoons vanilla.

Instructions:

The oven is preheated to 350°F. In a little bowl, combine the flour, cocoa powder, baking powder, and salt, and put in a safe spot. Pour the THC Oil and the cleaved chocolate into a double boiler over high heat.

As the water bubbles in the lower container, whisk the chocolate and oil until dissolved and smooth. Remove from heat and the corn syrup whisked in and also brown sugar, fruit purée. Mix in the egg whites and vanilla.

Beat the blend very well until smooth, at that point mix in the flour blend until very much fused. Oil a 9-by-13-inch heating skillet. Empty the hitter into the dish. Heat for 18 to 23 minutes, or until the focal point of the top is practically firm to the touch. Allow to cool.

Cannabis Brownies with Walnuts

Ingredients:

1c. of cannabis butter, 3c. of white sugar, 1 tbsp. of vanilla, 4 eggs, 1/2 c. flour, 1c. of powder unsweetened cocoa, 1 tsp. salt, 1c. of semisweet chocolate chips, 1 c. of sliced pecans

Instructions:

Preheat the stove to 175 degrees. Oil a baking dish, lightly. Join the liquefied cannabis butter, sugar, and vanilla in a big bowl. Beat in the eggs and mix altogether. Filter together the flour, cocoa powder, and salt.

Join the flour mixture into that of the chocolate steadily until it blends. Mix in the chocolate chips. The batter is then sprinkled equitably into the heating dish. Bake in the preheated stove for 40 minutes. Move the brownies from the oven and let it cool totally.

Sprinkle Brownies

Ingredients:

Canni bitter, 3 T water 1.4 lbs, chocolate chips, 6 eggs, ¾ tsp vanilla concentrate, 3c sugar, 1c flour, 1 T powder powder, ¾ tsp salt, 1 pkg. chocolate chips, 2 ½ oz. pretzels, 1 graham saltine pie crust, 1c butterscotch chips, 4c smaller than normal marshmallows

Instructions:

Preheat oven to 350 degrees and line skillet with parchment paper. Wish softened butter and chocolate chips over grill until liquefied and smooth.

The remaining baking ingredients should be added together and beat well. Empty batter into heating sheet and top with pretzels into batter, include crumbled graham wafer covering into hitter.

Prepare for 3-35 minutes. Add marshmallows and butterscotch and heat an additional 5 minutes 7. Remove let cool.

Canna-Chocolate Brownie Cake

Ingredients:

12 1 (18.25 ounce) packed devils food cake blend, 1 (3.9 ounce) instant chocolate pudding blend, 4 eggs, 1 cup acrid cream, 1/4 cup cannabis oil, ¼ cup vegetable oil, 1/2 cup water, 2 cups semisweet chocolate chips.

Instructions:

Preheat stove to 350 degrees F (175 degrees C). Oil and flour a 10-inch Bundt container. Have all ingredients at room temperature. In a huge bowl, mix together cake blend and that of the pudding.

Make a well in the inside and pour in eggs, sour cream, cannabis oil, vegetable oil, and water. Beat on low speed until mixed. Scratch bowl, and beat 4 minutes on medium speed. Mix in chocolate chips.

Empty batter into prepared dish. Bake in the preheated stove for 50 minutes to an hour, or until a toothpick inserted into the center of the cake comes out clean. Serve after cooling down.

Canna-Chocolate Butter Brownies

Ingredients:

15 1/4 cup cannabis butter, ¼ cup normal butter, 1/4 cup unsweetened cocoa, 1 cup water 2 cups sugar 2 cups universally handy flour, 1/2, teaspoon salt, 1/2 cup

buttermilk, 1 teaspoon baking soda, 2 eggs, beaten, 1 teaspoon vanilla concentrate, 3 drops red food coloring (optional).

Frosting: ½ cup butter or margarine, 1/4 cup unsweetened cocoa, 1/4 cup buttermilk, 1 pound confectioners' sugar, 1 teaspoon vanilla concentrate, Dash salt

Instructions:

In a pot, bring both cannabis and ordinary butter, cocoa and water to a bubble. Cool. In the meantime, in a big blending bowl, add sugar, flour and salt. Pour cocoa blend over dry ingredients; blend well. Mix buttermilk and baking soda; add to batter alongside eggs, vanilla, and food coloring whenever wanted.

Blend until very much mixed. Fill an oiled 15-in. x 10-in. x 1-in. lubed and floured baking container. Bake at 350 degrees F for 20 minutes. For icing, dissolve margarine, cocoa and buttermilk in a pot. Mix in sugar, vanilla and salt. Spread over warm cake. Top with nuts whenever wanted.

Canna-Carrot Cake

Ingredients:

4 eggs, 1/4 cups vegetable oil, 2 cups white sugar, 2 teaspoons vanilla concentrate, 2 cups universally handy flour, 2 teaspoons baking soda, 2 teaspoons baking powder,

1/2 teaspoon salt, 2 teaspoons ground cinnamon, 3 cups ground carrots, 1 cup cleaved walnuts

For Frosting : 1/4 cup cannabis butter, ¼ cup vegetable oil, 8 ounces cream cheddar, mellowed 4 cups confectioners' sugar, 1 teaspoon vanilla concentrate, 1 cup diced walnuts.

Instructions: Preheat oven to 350 degrees F (175 degrees C). Oil and flour a 9x13 inch dish. In a huge bowl, beat together eggs, oil, white sugar and 2 teaspoons vanilla. Blend in flour, baking soda and powder, salt and cinnamon. Mix in carrots. Crease in walnuts. Fill arranged skillet. Bake in the preheated stove for 40 to 50 minutes, or until a toothpick embedded into the center of the come out clean. Cool for 10 minutes, at that point turn out onto a wire rack and cool totally.

To Make Frosting: In a medium bowl, the two butter combined, cream cheese, confectioners' sugar and 1 teaspoon vanilla. Beat until the blend is smooth and velvety. Mix in cleaved walnuts. Frost the cooled cake.

Hash Oil Candy Bars

The hash oil mix can likewise be utilized to make a natural kind of candy bar as follows: Combine 1/2 cup each of slashed dates, raisins, figs, and ground almonds with 1 teaspoon each of ground aniseed, nutmeg and ginger. These can be warmed marginally and 4 tablespoons of the hot hashish/spread mix can be joined with the above ingredients. The blend is then cooled, kneaded or rolled, and cut into singular piece of candy. These might be wrapped separately in waxed paper, foil or plastic. Or on the other hand the ingredients can be joined with 1 cup of water, warmed also mixed, before blending in hash oil/butter. The blend is then warmed at a low temperature and mixed continually to forestall searing. At the point when this blend has thickened to a functional consistency, it is spread on a well greased baking tin and set in a oven at 22S"F for 30 minutes or until hard enough to cut into singular squares.

A portion of these candies being sold in the secret market come in printed wrappeu statina the specific measure of hash oil per bar. A few producers include a gram of powdered ginseng to each bar. The ginseng balances the mindboggling impacts of the sweets and encourages the consumer to keep up better under its impact.

Easy Candy Balls

This recipe requires no extraordinary arrangements of the cannabis material. It very well may be produced using plain cannabis, hashish or hash oil. Furthermore, it requires no cooking. The oils present in the nut butter fill in as a mechanism for the cannabis resins. Join '1-pound nut butter with 1 ounce or a greater amount of finely filtered cannabis, or 1/2 to 1 ounce of pummeled finely-shaved hashish, or 5 to 15 grams of hash oil.

Include a couple of tablespoons of honey as per your tooth sweetness. what's more, modest quantities of whatever else that satisfies: dried currants, diced coconut, ground orange or lemon strip, powdered cloves or nutnteg.

These ingredients are kneaded until completely mixed. Fold into singular balls about the size of a big marble. This ought to be wrapped independently in waxed paper, foil, or transparent wrap, and held under refrigeration to forestall the nut butter from getting malodorous. A couple of candy balls ought to be a ball.

Cannabis Milkshake (And Ice Cream Too)

Mix 1/2 ounce or a greater amount of finely-pummeled cannabis leaves and flowers (no seeds or stems) with 16 ounces of creamer (half cream and half milk). Include a level teaspoon of lecithin granules. Blend these in a blender for I or 2 minutes. Pour the substance of the blender into a pot and heat delicately for 10 minutes in a twofold boiler. Try not to overcook, or curds will isolate from the milk. Mix in a few tablespoons of nectar while the blend is hot.

Empty the blend into the blender container, include 1/2 teaspoon of vanilla concentrate, spread the top, and refrigerate for a few hours until chilled. At the point when you wish to drink it, put it on the electric blender again for 30 seconds and serve with straw in a glass.

In the event that you need to make it into ice cream or frozen yogurt, include a crude egg and whip completely in the blender until foamy. Fill any appropriate vessel, for example, an unfilled cheese or ricotta holder, or into singular custard cups.

Put a top on the holders, or spread the cups with waxed paper or plastic wrap and spot these in the cooler. Try not to stand by excessively well before freezing, or the whipped surface will settle to its unique liquid state.

In the event that you like, this dessert or shake can be made with hashish or hash oil. To do as such, first disintegrate hashish or hash oil in a small measure of butter. At that point add it to the half-and-half (half cream and half milk)/lecithin blend as in the past. A euphoric dessert can be made by covering this frozen yogurt with cannabis chocolate icing.

Cannabis Chocolate Icing

In the event that you smash a bud of newly dried cannabis between your fingers, you may perceive a chocolate-like smell blended among its aromas. There is no genuine likeness between cocoa beans and cannabis. The resemblance is just in our discernments. In any case, it is sufficient that a high evaluation of fragrant grass cultivated in Mexico is alluded to- at any rate in that nation - as chocolate. It is conceivable to exploit this inquisitive comparability and apply it in specific plans, for example, the following:

Melt 4 ounces of cannabis tar in a double boiler. Include one teaspoon or a greater amount of vanilla concentrate. While blending, include 4 ounces of honey. Altogether, mix the entirety of the ingredients.

You currently have an icing that can be utilized in recipes for bakery of your own choice or invention, for example, cannabis layer cake, iced cupcakes, stoned- - out dessert garnish; or you can simply spread it on crackers. It's so accursed finger-licking great that you may never at any point move beyond the finger-licking stage.

This icing tastes incredibly like chocolate icing, yet twenty minutes or so in the wake of eating it, you'll easily forget a chocolate cake that caused you to feel along these lines. A good variety can be made by including a teaspoonful of orange extract during the mixing.

Cannabis Butternut Squash Soup

Butternut squash is loaded with vitamin A, fiber and potassium. This soup is generous and will top you off just as is overflowing with flavor. It can undoubtedly turn into a velvety soup by including milk or cream.

Ingredients:

Butternut squash (3 lbs., seeds expelled and stripped), Vegetable oil (1 teaspoon), Red pepper (1, diced), Chicken stock (5 cups, low salt), Salt, Butter (1 tablespoon, unsalted), Onion (1, diced), Nutmeg, Black pepper, Sour cream, Cannabutter (1 ½ teaspoons).

Instructions:

Squash is cut into pieces and set aside until required. Heat a huge stock pot and liquefy butter alongside oil. At that point put in pepper, onion and salt to taste; cook for 8 minutes until onions are clear. Include stock and squash, mix and cook for 20 minutes until squash gets delicate.

If any squash remains, remove from pot and puree with some stock and then empty into pot. Include dark pepper, nutmeg and salt to taste at that point put in cannabutter and mix until spread melts for around 4 minutes. Serve, garnished with sour cream.

Creamy Cannabis Smoothie

Smoothies are very versatile and helpful, and you can try different things with numerous variations from this recipe by including various products of fruits and spices. At the point when you're ravenous yet don't want to prepare a major meal, smoothies can hold you over, however this specific smoothie may leave you feeling hungrier than when you began. Serve this chilly cool fruity cannabis infused treat on a hot day when turning the stove on is an excessive amount to shoulder.

Ingredients:

4 tablespoons Simple Cannabutter, 2 cups milk, ⅓ cup creamer, ½ cup plain yogurt, 1 banana, ½ cup new blueberries ½ cup new strawberries, 2 teaspoons honey, 6 ice shapes

Instructions:

In a sauté skillet, soften cannabutter over low heat. The softened butter should then be placed in the blender with the milk, creamer, yogurt, banana, blueberries, strawberries, and honey. Mix this blend until smooth (at any rate 1½ minutes in a powerful blender). At that point, with the blender running, drop in the ice cubes, each in turn, until the consistency is smooth.

Wake and Bake Smoothie

Smoothies are extraordinary for the individuals who need nourishment at any point. This smoothie is loaded up with sweetness and nutrients from fruits with included canna-oil to "boost" it.

Ingredients:

Banana (1), Almond milk (1/cup, unsweetened), Chia seeds (1 teaspoon), Frozen berries (1/2 cup), Canna-coconut oil (1 tablespoon, softened), Almonds (10, crude)

Instructions:

Put all Ingredients: into a blender and blend until smooth. Then serve that way or chill with ice before serving.

Almond Joy

Ingredients:

2 grams cannabis shake or bud, finely ground 7 liquid ounces coconut cream, ¼ cup chocolate syrup, 1 16 ounces almond milk Whipped cream, mint, and strawberries, to garnish.

Equipment: cheesecloth

Instructions:

The coconut cream is infused. You'll have to make what the French call a "bouquet garni," or an herb group, yet for this situation, "bouquet cannabis" would be the proper term. Pound your herb and enclose it by cheesecloth, tying the pack shut so you have a "tea sack." Make sure the string is sufficiently long to bind to the container's handle so you can recover the "bouquet cannabis" later.

Cook it gradually with the coconut cream in a little pan over an exceptionally low fire for about 2 hours, and as long as 4 hours if you have the opportunity. After the mixture is finished, expel the "bouquet cannabis" and dispose of.

Join the coconut cream with the chocolate syrup and almond milk. Shake in a shaker with ice. Strain and have it garnished with whipped cream, mint, and strawberries, whenever wanted.

Medical Cannabis Applesauce Pancake Recipe

Ingredients:

2 c. dry pancake mix, 1/2c. milk, 1c. apple sauce, 2 eggs, 1 tsp. cinnamon, ground 1 tsp. lemon juice, 1 cup Canna butter.

Instructions:

Turn on a skillet or frying pan that is delicately oiled to medium heat. By then get out a broad mixing bowl and mix the pancake mix and cinnamon.

In this mix, make a "pit" and in this hole, the eggs, milk, lemon crush, fruit purée should be added and blend until the consistency is smooth. Utilizing a scoop, pour the hitter onto the warmed iron or frying pan.

Fry until simply splendid cocoa on each side. Present with Canna butter and maple syrup or jam

Apple Chronic Tea

The advantages of apple juice are broad and can help in weight reduction; it is high in acidity and can help in managing diabetes. This is an extraordinary evening tea with a quieting impact.

Ingredients:

cannabis (1 bud), Captain Morgan's rum (1 shot), tea pack (1), hot apple cider.

Instructions:

Open the tea bag sachet and void substance. At that point, fill sachet with cannabis. Secure tea sack and put into a cup alongside cider and rum. Mix and cover permitting to soak for 10 minutes. In the event that tea isn't sufficiently warm, microwave rapidly, then serve.

CannaChoc Pudding

Give yourself or visitor a genuine upbeat time with this dessert. The use of fresh fruits is ideal as topping for this dish.

Ingredients:

Egg whites (2), cornstarch (2 tablespoons), canna butter (3 tablespoons, liquefied), vanilla (1 teaspoon), cocoa (10 tablespoons, unsweetened), whole milk (2 ¼ cups), Sugar (1/2 cup), raspberries.

Instructions:

Beat egg whites utilizing a blender. Mix cornstarch and cocoa then include 1 cup milk and rush until smooth. Heat extra milk alongside sugar and canna butter; whisk and cook for about 3 minutes. Put in cocoa blend and lower fire.

Whisk much of the time, then at that point take pan from fire and cool for 10 minutes. Include a cup of cooled blend to egg whites; whisk to mix it all up and afterwards, add to pan. Heat on a low fire.

Do not boil then remove from fire and put in vanilla. Set aside to cool. Refrigerate until chilled. Present with raspberries or any fresh fruit of your choice.

Canna-Mashed Potatoes

Ingredients:

6 medium chestnut potatoes, stripped and cubed, 1/2 cup warm milk, 1/4 cup cannabis butter, 3/4 teaspoon salt, Dash pepper

Instructions:

Place potatoes in a pan and cover with water. Cover and heat to the point of boiling; cook for 2025 minutes or until extremely soft. Drain water well. Include milk, cannabis butter, salt and pepper; pound until light and fluffy.

Canna-Creamy Potato Salad

Ingredients:

5 red potatoes, 5 Yukon Gold potatoes, 2 tablespoons cannabis butter salt and pepper to taste, 1/2 cup mayonnaise, 1/2 cup prepared mustard, 1/2 cup sour cream, 1 stem celery, finely diced 1 red onion, finely diced 2 little sweet pickles, finely shredded 1 green ringer pepper, cleaved cube and peel potatoes.

Ingredients:

Place potatoes in an enormous pan and have it covered with water. Cook over medium heat until potatoes are soft. Drain and put cooked potatoes in a big bowl. Pound potatoes with cannabis butter and salt and pepper to taste.

Once crushed, mix in the mayonnaise, mustard and sour cream. Mix continuously. Pour in the celery, onion, pickles and green pepper. Serve warm or at room temperature.

Sesame Mushroom Bourguignon

This dish has an Asian and French combination with a red wine sauce, substantial mushrooms and cannabis with umami. This dish will satisfy anybody that is fortunate to get a taste whether veggie lover or meat lovers.

Ingredients:

(4 tablespoons) Olive canna-oil, Earth balance stick butter (2 tablespoons), Cremini mushrooms (1 lb., cut), Carrot (1, stripped and minced), Scallions (3 tablespoons, cleaved), Garlic (3 cloves, diced), Vegetable stock (2 ¼ cups, natural), Yeast (1 ½ tablespoons), Sea salt, Sesame seeds (1 tablespoon, toasted), Black pepper, Olive oil (1 tablespoon), Sesame oil (2 teaspoons), Portobello mushrooms (1 lb., cut), Pearl onions (1 cup), Onion (1, cut), Thyme (2 teaspoons, slashed), Red wine (1 ½ cups, full bodied), Tomato glue (2 tablespoons, natural), Whole wheat flour (1 ½ tablespoons), Quinoa (2 cups, cooked)

Ingredients:

Soften half of butter alongside olive oil in a large Dutch oven over a medium fire. Sauté onions with a touch of pepper and salt. Mix and cook for 15 minutes until caramelized at that point expel from skillet and set aside until required. Raise fire and add ¼ cup stock to dish then 1 tablespoon of canna-oil. Put in onions and mushrooms and not many at once and cook until they start to get darkened marginally. Remove from skillet and set aside until required. Lower fire and include 2 tablespoons canna-oil at that point put in scallion, carrot, thyme and add pepper and salt to taste.

Cook for 10 minutes, at that point, put in garlic and cook for an extra 2 minutes. Include red wine and use spoon to scratch pot. Cook until wine has decreased considerably then placed in stock and glue alongside mushrooms and onions. Mix to join and bring to boil then put in yeast and remaining canna-oil.

Cook for 15 minutes. Blend flour in with extra butter and mix into stew. Put in sesame oil and cook for 10 minutes until stew gets thick; add pepper and salt to taste varying. Has it served with quinoa and top with sesame seeds?

CHAPTER SIX: CANNABIS EXTRACTIONS AND INFUSIONS

Infusions are the central core, the structure hinders, of incredible cannabis food. Each cook has his or her strategy, refined from long periods of experimentation. THC and CBD are two important components involves in the extraction and activation of cannabinoids; an important plant component, however, logical principles apply.

The rationale behind the extraction of edible cannabinoids is of science, which is simple. Naturally, THC-A and CBD-A particles are fat soluble that combine with fats (oils, margarine, milk, honey) and alcohols when heated.

The cannabinoid is a fat extract. THC and CBD are converted to THC-A and CBD-A when reasonably heated, conveying improved treats once gathered in the plant's trichomes. The basic of all techniques for extraction involve either getting the treats out of the cellulose cell wall or removing the material, and abandoning the skeletal cellulose.

The specialty of infusions is somewhat messier, as this form of specialty will be, generally. Everybody has their own peculiar means of achieving it. No means is correct or wrong so long as you follow some essential rules.

You can utilize a slow cooker, a hot plate, a skillet on the oven, or the broiler. You can either imbue it quick, or let it simmer for quite a long time (as long as you watch it cautiously and don't allow it to be consumed with heat). As is consistently the situation with cannabis (and a wonderful thing), the best way to discover the infusion that works best for you is to attempt a couple.

To prepare consumable extraction, cannabis is warmed tenderly in a fat or alcohol to separate cannabinoids that's fat soluble in nature. Infusions concentrated on was made utilizing liquor, butter, oil, milk, and honey, which isn't actually a fat yet a decent specialist for cannabinoid's suspension on the grounds that they're the ones used by culinary experts.

The means of carrying it out range from crude to cutting edge techniques. Some individual stuffs jars loaded with plant material and oil and then lay them down in a window where sunshine act on it to accomplish the work. Others utilizes a Magical Butter machine that concentrates, blends, and keeps up temperature parity and carries out extractions in 60 minutes. The two acts reported euphoric outcomes.

Majority of experts are some place in the middle of, adhering strictly to similar rules: cook moderate and low, allocating adequate time for the cannabinoids and terpenes to mix and simultaneously prevent the temperature from elevating so high to the point of dissipating the cannabinoids and terpenes (around 180- 220 degrees Fahrenheit).

Some experts tenderly simmer cannabis blossoms in margarine for a few days over low heat to separate cannabinoids and flavor, and others lets blossoms or trims mix in with the coconut oil in an extremely low oven for at least eight to about ten hours. places cannabis and oil can also be placed in an indestructible glass container putting it in a half loaded crockpot with water and applied low heat for six-eight hours.

This regulates the temperature, as some crockpots get excessively hot even on their most reduced settings and can consume the infusion. Hash can be utilized for individual infusions yet a strategy that beckon on simmering cannabis in water can be applied, having a diminish breaking point than butter or oil, to forestall consuming.

A cannabis-infused item will likely be created that is as near the first as conceivable by gradually extracting cannabinoids without an excess of warmth. It is possible that margarine loses its consistency in the extraction procedure, but in cooking, it is not feasible to work out. With use on cookies, it won rise and will level out, and you won't be able to prepare hollandaise sauce with it. You need to have the option to utilize your margarine and oils a similar way any mixture is made.

Flavor

Infusing cannabis with oil and margarine produce a bitter, home grown taste that is ideal and extremely, just portrayed as "green." No culinary modifier's is available for cannabis flavor; "Natural" is the abused term utilized in the absence of the language to depict the plant's profundity.

Not so long, majorities of cannabis culinary experts tried to conceal the cannabis taste by using solid flavors so that burger joints could use it without perceiving the real taste. That is art in itself and, once more, a profoundly close to individual's decision.

A couple of recipes was included that totally cover the cannabis taste consequently. But as the cannabis showcase opens up, giving culinary specialists a practically boundless palette of cannabis "flavors" to work with, cannabis is now regarded as a significant flavoring, straight up there with oregano, basil, and tarragon.

Culinary experts relatively use cannabis enhances in like manner in which painters uses shading and performers uses notes. The cannabis in some infusion includes subtle flavor much as an experiment on basil-mixed olive oil did.

Some experts cherish the flavor of the plant; being baffled with cannabis cooking, not long ago in light of the fact that sugar-loaded desserts intended to shroud the cannabis flavor did not create any sense of appeal to anyone. Concealing the flavor, as claimed, enhances excessive consumption.

At the point when that brownie tastes so great, it's anything but difficult to overlook that it's additionally getting you high which keeps somewhat "green" flavor, just as shading.

Most specialists cooking with cannabis esteem the plant's position in their collection, a mending herb with a solid taste profile much the same as turmeric or garlic (with a psychoactive bend). For some experts, the use of cannabis for cooking as the same resemblance with blending a martini with spirits of great quality.

It is like the need to taste the gin or vodka. It's the equivalent with cannabis, and that is the distinction between cooking with cannabis and being a gourmet expert with cannabis. You always have the flavor.

Blossoms and Sugar Leaves

In the process of cannabinoid's extraction from blossoms and the minuscule "sugar leaves" that are cut off when flowers are trimmed (otherwise called "manicure") is the widely recognized technique for making infusions mostly known.

Flowers contain more trichome included and make a stronger mixture with more predictable outcomes than trim. Blossoms additionally bestow a more grounded home grown flavor. In light of the fact that sugar leaves have more chlorophyll, they also taste bitter. Utilize dried flowers and sugar leaves for infusions.

For most strategies, the blossoms and leaves must be finely grinded. This should be possible utilizing a coffee processor, a mortar and pestle, or a fine work screen. The screen should be positioned over a plate and utilize your hands to mix the flowers and leaves on the screen (don gloves; it will be clingy) to crush them finely into a powder.

Decarboxylation

Decarboxylation is the way toward warming cannabis to actuate THC and CBD. Decarboxylation has been subjected to hot discussions ever since the US government specialists founded out in 1970 that warming cannabis to around 200 degrees Fahrenheit severs THC-A and CBD-A carboxyl radicals and expands THC and CBD rate which makes cannabis unmistakably increasingly powerful.

A few culinary experts accept decarboxylation to be in consistency and essential when cannabis is cooked and making of tinctures. Some avoid the progression altogether, considering it to be an exercise in futility that might disintegrate important mixes. Next to zero vaporization of cannabinoids and terpenes happens if the temperature stays beneath 246 degrees Fahrenheit.

Most specialists try not to decarboxylate cannabis before making oil and butter infusions since that extraction procedure adequately warms the cannabis to change over THA-A into THC. To either decarb or not is profoundly close to individuals' inclinations.

Cannabis is consistently decarded by some experts prior to the production of oils, margarines, or tinctures, since, it is claimed to just appear to work. This shows that a decent high is appreciated and furthermore acknowledges that CBD, which is likewise discharged all the while, improve sleep. To actuate CBD, the oven is regulated somewhat higher and lets the cannabis heat for an additional fifteen minutes. The basic procedure of warming blossoms in a stove pack follows.

You will require:

- Oven bag

- Oven safe dish

- Entire cannabis flowers and additionally sugar trim leaves

Instructions:

Preheat oven. To actuate THC, put the stove at 250°F. To initiate CBD, increase the stove to 275°F. Put cannabis in oven bag and move out all the air.

A tie should be knotted to seal the pack. Place sack into oven safe dish and put in center of preheated stove.

To initiate THC, set at 250°F and heat for at least 30 minutes. To initiate CBD, set at 275°F, and heat for a minimum of 45 minutes. Take away from the stove and allow cooling down totally. You can place the pack in the cooler to accelerate the procedure.

Oil and Butter Extractions

Each cook has a somewhat unique strategy for infusing oil and margarine, yet most follow a similar general rules. You can utilize anyplace from a quarter to an ounce of trim or flowers per quarter pound of butter or quarter-cup of oil and once more, this proportion is exceptionally close to home.

The ratio of cannabis to fat in direct proportion legitimately influences the infusion's strength, which likewise to a great extent relies upon the cannabis quality, age, and state utilized. Infusions will probably contrast from bunch to clump except if you can get the cannabis tried.

The optimal way to oil and butter mixtures is to cook them low and moderate, ideally at roughly 200 degrees Fahrenheit. Temperatures over 350 degrees Fahrenheit provoke unpredictable oils and terpenes to dissipate, and the fats to be consumed.

Watch out for the margarine or oil as it simmers, mix sporadically, and utilize a sweets thermometer in case you're stressed over it getting excessively hot. At the point when Cannabis Olive Oil, some slight bubbling is allowed to simmer and mixed for the whole time the oil is heated. It's the same in preparing any food. In the event that it's burnt, it's burnt.

In a way, that is a costly mix-up in light of the fact that you've recently consumed an ounce of cannabis. For this explanation, numerous experts present water, which has a lower boiling point compare to margarine or oil (212 degrees Fahrenheit), into the procedure. Water regulates the temperature, keeping the fat and cannabis from being consumed with heat, and furthermore ingests chlorophyll, which adds to cannabis green color, smell and taste.

Improvement is observed in few. For the individuals who need chlorophyll's blood-oxygenating impacts, that is a drawback. Whatever technique you employ, green oil or margarine is inevitable provided you implant it with blossoms and sugar leaves. Contingent upon the crude materials you utilize, the final item will fall in-between lime green to woodland green, practically earthy colored.

Hash Infusions

Hash, intense with sap trichomes, when utilized holds few advantages compare to plant material in many imbuements. One has advantages involves dissolving straightforwardly into oil or margarine, wiping out the need to strain out cannabis particles and manage untidy cheesecloth.

The procedure likewise expels the small hairs on the plant, which can pose difficulty for individuals with intestinal tract issues to process. Utilizing hash rather than plant material additionally takes out the green tone and a significant part of the home-grown flavor. Hash is way stronger than blossoms and sugar leaves.

A few grams of hash in a stick of spread or four ounces of oil makes a gentle imbuement, and commonly the gram's norm ranges from three to five, yet everything relies upon the cannabis power. Hash can be bought in pharmacy and retail locations, however, not all hash is made equivalent.

The extraction of hash inappropriately with butane has a probability of adding to your food. For the most advantageous and most secure outcomes, search for bubble hash or dry filter. You can prepare your own hash contained in ice water, however, suggestion in doing so in not without getting your work done or finding a decent instructor.

Regardless of the information you have been exposed with in the past, avoid making your hash with butane. It's hazardous and unhealthy to a great deal, and a few districts in states where cannabis is lawful are now prohibiting the training.

CHAPTER SEVEN: REGULATORY INTERVENTIONS ON CANNABIS FOOD INTAKE

DOSAGE AND POTENCY RATIO

There are various means, by which cannabis mixed nourishments can be produced, and there are boundless structures and diversities of cannabis accessible to work with, without no doubt, there is need to adequate plan on your dosing, also test each new bunch under regulated measures occurring, prior to the extension to friends for use.

The euphoric, far reaching, and blissful impacts of cannabis result from super material utilized sensibly and moderately. This is vital as seen with the different psyche delicacies. The unaccustomed regulations develop the most fulfilling feelings ever. Should you consider cannabis early and late in the day, at that point the utilization of cannabis turns into a dulling propensity, and as time goes by, creates torpidity and distraction. In any case, utilized sparingly, once in a while, and in happy conditions, cannabis builds joy.

Dosing is significantly important to cannabis cooking and numerous individuals are generally inquisitive about the subject of cannabis. Dosing is central to the strength of the medication and patient's situation and size. There are three various means to regulate the drug strength and the effect of the final cannabis-mixed foods:

- Modify the measure of plant material utilized in the margarine, oil, or tincture as indicated by the nature of the cannabis and relying upon the piece of the plant you are utilizing; bud, bloom, leaf trim, or shake;

- Change the quality of the cannabis butter, oil, tincture, or flour utilized in the formula;

- Modify the size of the food per servings

Begin with surveying the strength of your mystery ingredient before estimating the proportion of cannabis to margarine required to make up your recipe. It ranges from five to ten grams of the best hashish to produce an exceptionally strong strain, sufficient to be infused into a pound of spread, however, when you're utilizing low-strength cut leaves, a minimum of two ounces or a greater amount of leaf to be mixed in a similar measure of margarine. The cannabis buds should be dried and thoroughly mix with a decent dependable guideline being about an ounce of cannabis to a pound of margarine.

There are numerous self-factors that can go into building up the correct measurements for you or your patient which includes weight (two persons cannot require the same amount; a heavier person would require more), digestion (how your body utilizes nourishments and the synthetic compounds in cannabis determines the impact on your body system), and dietary patterns (consuming cannabis on a vacant stomach will have a greater impact). Appropriately dealing with your dosing can assist you with in dealing with your medication. There is uniqueness pertaining to each patient, having a clear understanding of self-limits and requesting for assistance to keep up a constant dosing.

Eating an excessive amount of cannabis can bring about languor, inability to focus, elevated pulse or circulatory strain, and elation of happiness. If you perceive you may have consumed excessively, do not panic and relax. Cannabis is non-harmful, so it won't have any enduring or deadly impacts. The side effects will go away in a couple of hours. Ensure you drink plenty of water and avoid a drug containing food until the side effects fade away.

In case you're opportune to have access to a rich flow of cannabis, a little experimentation will let you know the right dosing for your body. To achieve a great outcome, make a numerous smaller bud and preserve it in a refrigerator. This can be helpful to maintain a constant dose before a new dosage is tried on.

In the event that a recipe you'd prefer requires a bigger measure of mixed spread or oil than you to regard savvy, basically weaken the intensity of the cannabutter from your cooler by including non-mixed lined margarine. Remember that clinical patients may require a more powerful dose than healthier people, which is dependent upon their condition.

The consumption of cannabis makes you feel some physical symptoms; elevated pulse, dizziness, difficulty in breathing, you experience excessive mouth dryness, and your response is reduced. You feel anxious and paranoid, hallucinating for hours like you've been walking miles, lack of orientation to time, event, and you have thought like a dying man.

The rate of mortality is not as a result of excessive consumption of cannabis as it does not affect body cells and organs. However, increase in cannabis users is seen and a resultant in frequent emergency cases.

Excessive consumption of cannabis is an emergency. The impacts go from mush cerebrum (don't eat cannabis edibles before occasions where it's inevitable to meet notable individuals) to approach mental shock. Your psyche is sluggish, creaky, with profound winds and plunges just like a wooden rollercoaster.

Overdosing with food containing cannabis makes you strange in social gathering; however, is a lot better way than bringing down such a large number of martinis. You'll have a head loaded with various thoughts and interconnections, the following day, yet you won't need to stress over past actions or words. You stated, "Can I simply rest on the lounge chair?" And that is practically what you did.

Finding Your Dose

The difficulty in the standardization of natural medications has led to the removal of cannabis from pharmacopoeia long before it was banned. A tablespoon of cannabis margarine (for the most part thought to be one portion) can differ uncontrollably in strength from another tablespoon.

With such a significant number of factors, the dosage of cannabis in food is chaotic with science estimations. It's in reality, there is more to just an art. When a new cluster of oil or butter is made, bio-assay, which is a form of assessment, biologically, carried out to gauge the effects of a substance, is performed.

For each serving, some broad rules were followed for the measure of cannabis utilized. A lower quality of flower, with a third of a gram and hash of sixth gram provokes panic attacks in considerably large number of people.

However, every cluster interprets that contrastingly and each individual's affectability is unique. THC includes in cannabis infusions is a factor, in any event, when precisely the same recipe is followed with exactness. The use of bio-examination is the best way to ascertain cannabis food influences on you in the absence of independent testing. Maintain a diary of implantations and plans that you've tried.

Record the date, time, cultivar, and where you bought or developed and gathered it, the amount you expended, and how it impacted you. A pattern will be drawn overtime to show how various cultivars and infusions impacts, and furthermore how tremendously unique each bunch can be.

Calculating dosage

The estimations of THC and CBD are done in milligrams. The cannabis amount of THC is with great variation, and to ascertain the amount of milligrams in cannabis is not feasible except when subjected to free testing. With respect to ten percentage of THC containing cannabis which form the basis on which THC is been calculated, and this is the general accepted standard by industry without normalization. The calculation of THC content is dependent on this normal can be useful when looking at plans yet, this won't be a secure sign of how strong a dish will be.

The estimations are likened to personal duty directions. When a gram of dried cannabis is weighted, it is equivalent to one thousand milligrams. A ten percentage of one thousand is equivalent to one hundred milligram which implies that one hundred milligrams of THC is found in a gram of cannabis at all time. You can compute the THC composition in a mixture by isolating the absolute number of milligrams in the formula by the quantity of cups it yields.

You would then be able to compute the level of THC in plans by duplicating the quantity of cups of spread or oil in the formula by the amount of THC in the imbuement. To estimate the amount per serving, the total content of THC in the whole dish is divided by the serving's number

Recommended doses

The standard portion for each serving is equivalent to 10 milligrams according to Colorado Cannabis Enforcement Division's, and this is in contrast to many persons-one bottles of beer, glass of wine, or mixed drink. The number's still unreasonably high for the Council with regards to cannabis regulations with a suggestion of five milligrams to newbie on cannabis consumption.

For certain individuals, it's of great comfort to consume THC of about ten milligrams while this amount (10 milligrams) seems high for first time users to consume. If you are uncomfortable with excessive intoxication, do you really have put yourself at risk?

Pause

The preparation of food, the sort of infusion, what the food is combined with, the amount you have consumed, all play significant roles on the impact of cannabis on the body after ingestion. Greasy, protein-rich nourishments escalate the impacts, sugar makes a quicker dispersion more rapidly, and liquor can aggravate the impacts and provoke distrustfulness. In combination with individual's digestion, body size and mass, individual natural chemistry, age, and resilience, and you have a convoluted arrangement of factors that make it difficult to know how and when the impacts of cannabis food will hit everyone at the table.

Every other person during supper could be laughing and settling all the more cheerfully into their seats while you feel indifferent. Hours could pass by. The compulsion to snatch one more chomp, particularly when the food prepared with cannabis is awesome, and this can be wild. The results can be humiliating, best case scenario, shocking at the very least, and keep going for quite a long time, even into the following day.

At this point where it's conveyed through food, it can take the cannabis can take at least two hours or more to settle in. After the cannabis has settled in, you can add a couple more snacks and these increases in three fold the whammy. A newbie to cannabis food should ingest small quantity initially and avoid having another afterwards. When there's no occurrence, you should appreciate delectable food and it's not the apocalypse. Eat somewhat more next time.

Not created equal

Except if you've just attempted a cannabis dish in the past or have your cannabis tried for THC content, you can't anticipate how it will influence you regardless of your resistance. There is a probability for differences to exists between ounces of different grower. Power, influenced by ecological components, developing conditions, and hereditary qualities, shifts even in a cultivar with precisely the same hereditary qualities as another developed at an alternate time by a similar cultivator. Put into consideration, any food prepared with cannabis that hasn't been freely tried for potency, and consumes it. You can test the cannabis on yourself but modest quantity should be used. Never depend on another person's sentiment.

Start low, go slow

In particularly, when you're encircled by the odor of warm scones directly from the broiler, it can pose some difficulty, however, to abstain effectively from over-inebriation is to begin with a sample segment of cannabis food and hold up two hours or more to perceive what occurs. When trying to serve cannabis infused food, for example, cake or brownies to beginner cannabis eaters, it is recommended that you begin with pieces generally the size of their thumb cushions.

There is also a suggestion of moving toward cannabis nourishments as you would 100-proof (or more) liquor. Start out by sipping. If you gulp a container of tequila, you'll have a horrendous day. Something very similar applies. Some start individuals by providing cannabis food with toppings, little dishes of soup, or little tidbits. It is highly unlikely anybody can eat a whole feast. You cannot go through it else, you would find yourself in coma.

Infusion of cannabis in food that can be added widely to different dishes permits everybody to be answerable for their own fate during supper, and that is critical. Prepare non-mixed adaptations to give visitors to prevent them from been enticed by the look and odor of food not meant for them. When you consume excessive cannabis, there is no change of decision. The likelihood of doing it again is slim after your initial experience that once. Why get yourself through it by any stretch of the imagination?

Controlling the medicinal potency of marijuana foods

In early discussion, you can remember that the three different ways to control the therapeutic strength and the effect of the completed cannabis nourishments:

- change the measure of plant material utilized in the margarine, oil, or tincture as indicated by the nature of the cannabis and relying upon the piece of the plant bud, bloom, leaf trim, or shake you are utilizing,

- alter the quality of the cannabis spread, oil, tincture, or flour utilized in the formula

- modify the size in which the food is served.

Modifying for Marijuana Quality

The cannabis nature utilized in the production of spread, oil, tincture, or flour, have an impact on the intensity of the final food products. In comparison, an ounce of great and low-grade cannabis, the high grade possesses a greater number of essentials ingredients. You should often utilize high grade clinical cannabis, yet rely on accessible cannabis; the measure of cannabis can be expanded or diminished as needs be.

You can utilize tactile strategies to assist better with the understanding whether to utilize pretty much cannabis to coke the extracts. Should the medication look unremarkable, needs smell, isn't resinous to handling, similar stale taste, has restricted impacts, or needs newness, all things considered, utilizing more cannabis will be increasingly valuable.

The cannabis is considered to be of high grade when it's contained, all the necessities, therefore, the highest therapeutic effects can be demonstrated with a typical or lower amount. The simple approaches to utilize your faculties to recognize high- and poor-quality cannabis are;

- Sight: Are there noticeable trichomes (resinous crystal-like arrangements)? Does it look stained or aged? You can utilize an amplifying gadget to inspect the material to note the inherent quality.

- Smell: Is the plant material pungent and ready, or does it need fragrance or smell to some degree of stale? Is there a smelly smell? New, good quality cannabis has a unique scent.

- Contact: Does the material have a clingy pitch when scoured between your fingers? Is it a white inclination (fine buildup), or does it have a coarse surface?

- Taste: When smoked or disintegrated does the cannabis have a chemical or aroma taste? Does it taste new or stale? Is the taste ground-breaking or powerless?

- Impact: When smoked or disintegrated does medication that have a solid and quick impact, or does it take more than typical to be sufficiently cured?

- Freshness: old medication or inappropriately stored medication may encounter a breakdown of cannabinoids. Disintegrating, over-dried, or stained cannabis could be an indication of absence of it being fresh.

Utilizing Buds, Flowers, Leaf Trim, or Shake to Control Strength

In an attempt to produce a suitable extract for cooking to often bring about the ideal impact, it is pertinent to understand how the key role of the ratio of cannabis buds to its leaf. However, this is not a definite science in light of the fact that each cannabis plant is unique, the people at Steep Hill Labs in California who test medication for patient cooperatives in the state, check that on normal, the leaves or trimmings from a cannabis plant are about twenty-five percent as solid as buds or blossoming bunches from a similar plant.

This implies that generally, a proportion of one to four of bud/blossom to leaf trim or shake will create comparable restorative impacts. In the event that you are utilizing the buds/flowers of the plant you should just use from a quarter ounce of buds/flowers to an ounce of leaf trim or shake; or on a bigger size of more vulnerable pot, utilize one ounce of bud/blossoms to a quarter pound of leaf trim or shake. This ratio of one to four is the general proportion that ought to give a moderately steady outcome.

Decreasing the Plant Material Flower Potency

In the event that you need reduced strength, other choice to consider is to include less plant material than is called for in the extraction recipe to make a less intense mixture for cooking. This is a decent technique in situations where you can't get hold of enormous amounts of cannabis. Making margarine, oil, or tincture with small amounts of cannabis may likewise be alluring provided that you need to prepare dinners for a gathering of patients or appreciate bigger parts or any mix of bites, soups, starters, sides, courses, or treats. Altering the weed strength spread, oils, and tinctures, will assist you with having a superior encounter, and thus will help to cultivate wellbeing. Often consider with caution the side effects.

Titration for Optimal Affect

When the recipe is prepared, your last opportunity to meddle with the medication strength is by manipulating the size of the food part. Here, titration technique is of the essence. In medical sciences, titration deals with modifying the different portions of the drugs or substance until the ideal affect is accomplished.

Titration gives room for patients to figure out which measure of certain restorative nourishments sufficiently sedate, without overpowering and excessive dosing. In a situation whereby uncertainty exists in relation to how much prescription needed by you, despite the fact that you adequately modified the formula by the measure of plant material included and the measure of cannabis oil utilized, you can decide on the amount of food to be consumed.

At the point when a patient with no experience is presented with a new regimen containing food, such patient should commence by ingesting a little segment of the food and observe up to an hour before looking at the effects. By then you can evaluate the requirement for pretty much medication. In an important situation, ingest other segment of the food and hold up an additional for about thirty to sixty minutes.

You can increase your food consumption when your condition needs more drugs. After some time, you will start to precisely decide what segment size of specific nourishments function admirably for your clinical needs. You will be knowledgeable about the amount of food that increases your comforts. You will feel the help from this brilliant medication at its ideal quality for you. Utilize practical insight and caution while attempting new cured nourishments.

CHAPTER EIGHT: COOKING WITH CANNABIS: ADOPTING SAFETY MEASURES

The use of cannabis for cooking should be carried out by ensuring safety and should be done in a reasonable way. In other to prevent sickness as a result of ingested food on a norm, requires you to sustain precautionary measures. Cooking with cannabis is not different from food cooking therefore, maintain the same level of diligence and put into consideration the impacts it's likely to have on both the users and cannabis cook expert.

One way to be certain about having a great experience and prevent subsequent issues is to adequately review plant to be utilized, putting in place standardized safety measures, thoroughly learning, sharp mindfulness, and a lead of duty. There are consequences that arise when cannabis is utilized in unsafe manners therefore, it is essential to be aware of the fundamental safety measures to be observed during preparation and in handling of cannabis.

Safety Inspecting Marijuana

When you newly begin cooking with cannabis, it is critical to investigate the medication being utilized for indications of tainting. Natural contaminants, synthetic contaminants, and even maladies can be presented in cannabis. Under no circumstances should a plant material contaminated with quantifiable degrees of pesticides or fungicides be utilized.

Also, substance like powdery mildew should not be utilized despite not to be proven to cause diseases in human. Preventing rushing and adequately inspect the cannabis before cooking can assist with recognizing and maintain a strategic distance from undesirable tainting of your clinical nourishments. Ideally, it is beneficial to know the wellspring of the drug to have a superior thought of the development procedure.

Having the knowledge as regarding how cannabis is cultivated and stored will give you the clue on the standard employed in sanitary, the type of pesticides utilized and if it is likely to be contaminated with an active substance. Ordinarily you don't have a clue where the cannabis was developed, and that is alright. You can assess the cannabis for issues and avoid potential risk before cooking to help guarantee if it safe to be used by client. Here are some normal weed contaminants and how to remember them.

- **Mold and Mildew**

    Contagious developments, for example, mildews and molds, can be found on cannabis. Ideally all food and plants would be without mold, however when making therapeutic nourishments it is extra essential to be diligent. White fine mildew is tragically normal. This shows in a white fine substance on the leaf and flower surfaces that feels pasty rather than clingy.

You might have the option to distinguish other contagious issues by smell; the plant material may have smelly odor. At the point when the material is new, it can feel somewhat vile, and that is superior to dry and pale. A mold spores maybe found on the surface of a dried plant material. Dull staining can be an indicative sign that cannabis has been made impure with spores.

Utilize an amplifying gadget or magnifying lens to investigate probable contaminated issues. When a mold is placed under a magnifying lens, it appears as a thinning thread only distinctive in the part containing the growing spores, the head.

Cannabis contain a reasonable level of molds that's not harmful to the body but, an immune compromised person should avoid such as they already have a weakened immune system and might not be able to resist a little provoke by the mold. As suggested by the American Nursing Association, any plant material containing cannabis can be heated for about thirty minutes with a temperature of about 325° and still be able to preserve the THC which distil off at 380°.

You need not to worry about losing the active substance as the heat will kill quite some of the molds but not all due to differences in temperature required to kill different forms of molds. You should boil your cannabis to a reasonable extent to prevent yourself from developing health exacerbation by molds.

Uses of Pesticides and Fertilizers

For a while now, the cultivation of cannabis has not received adequate attention. Accordingly, individuals frequently utilize plant containing hazardous and brutal pesticides or additives. Some of the developed substances should not be utilized due to their hazardous properties. To identify contaminated plant is not an easy task but a simple tasting of a small portion of the leaf can show if there is residue of chemical present. Also, leaf discoloration might be an indicative sign that a plant is not healthy.

If you know pesticides to be risky to your health, it is pertinent to use cannabis of unidentified sources with extreme caution. Homemade packs for testing are available for you to use if you are worried to screen for some frequent toxins. Under no instance should you make use of quantifiable degrees of pesticides or fungicides if found on plant material.

Diseases and Pathogens

Cannabis plant has no exceptions to biological and pathogens issues that often plaque plants generally. If there is failure in the process of cultivating and handling, there is a high chance to be contaminated with pathogens that are injurious to the human body, and are not suitable for consumption. Color changes and taste can be used to identify some pathogens present on the leaf or plant surface. Should you have doubt about the safety of any cannabis plant, you should discard it with no delay.

BASIC COOKING SAFETY

You can commence cooking immediately you have ascertained that your cannabis is safe for use. Kitchen has its set standard to be followed to avoid contamination and to have a hygienic food safe for consumption. The preparation of cannabis containing food needs an extra attention to ensure its hazard free.

Cleanliness

The principal thing is to keep up a spotless and clean kitchen. Continuously, spotless before starting a task, during planning, and after completing that venture. Utilize safe and non-poisonous cleaning arrangements and prepare food on nonporous surfaces. All surface, sink territories, and materials ought to be cleaned and equipment ought to be in decent shape. The main process by which food is contaminated is inability to appropriately ensure cleanliness. It is your obligation to ensure your food readiness and cooking territories are kept clean to the maximum.

Dedicated Work Area

While you are getting ready restorative foods, your area of food preparation ought to be devoted distinctly to making therapeutic food sources. Individuals, pets, things, and food not identified with the preparation of clinical nourishments ought to be expelled from the territory. You need not a split attention during the preparation of cannabis foods; therefore, it is imperative to evacuate any potential interruptions before working with the cannabis. You might want to make your cooking to be fun, do so without compromising kitchen safety.

Hygiene

Ensure hand cleanliness at all time through hand washing with soap and warm water prior to when you handle your food. Make certain to keep sanitation guidelines even when your gear and utensils are being washed with your hands. By doing this you can prevent to the minimum transmission of microscopic organisms or natural contaminants to the foods.

Safety Equipment

Safety materials such as gear, similar to plastic or latex with no powder used in handling food, and a head covering, to maintain a strategic distance from tainting of the food should be utilized. Nobody appreciates finding a stray of hair in their dish, it is essential to take the right precaution when you cook outside your home for others. The only way to prevent allergic reaction to food contamination for some Individual is to ensure you adhere to sanitary guidelines.

Education

Almost all the states have courses developed on how to observe sanitation. It is an added advantage to take a course when you are cooking for others to know the accepted temperature, sanitary standards, diseases related to food, different allergens and cross-defilement.

Storage

Continuously preserve cannabis in a cool and dry environment to prevent heat form causing it to lose some of its properties, and avoid storing in a container at close proximity to the oven or over the fridge. You should be certain to keep away from inquisitive individuals the cannabis extractions and foods.

In other to avoid mixing up, ensure to name clearly all medication, spreads, oils, tinctures, and sedated nourishments. It is applicable to drugs containing food the same way we ensure children cannot get a hold of a bottle of pills. Read the label for instructions on proper storage and also take note of the half-life to ensure its freshness.

Other Safety Applications

The law identified illicit drug to be illegal and should you be found wanting, it can lead to loss of assistance on housing and school finances or might as well leads to loss of job. The consumption comes with a risk as long as the law does not identify it to be legal. It is up to you to make a decision if you can live up with this risk. Whereas, in states where cannabis it's lawful, it's a controlled substance and ought to be treated with a similar regard and attention that you would provide for liquor or doctor prescribed drugs. Store it out of reach of kids, and lock it up if need be.

It is prohibited consuming cannabis and driving simultaneously. Similarly, likewise with liquor and physician endorsed drug, it is risky and unlawful to eat cannabis while driving. Colorado and Washington have a cutoff point legally backed for the amount of cannabis in a driver's blood, and they are implementing them. Cannabis can stay up for as long as five hours. Avoid driving after you've eaten cannabis food.

There should be a clear label on the cannabis bottle to prevent accidental dosing to you, aged person, and nanny in the house. The label on the cannabis bottle should be clear and bold to denote its content.

Keep out of reach of pets, it's too much for them to handle. Get cannabis food far from pets, and it's quite expensive treat pets intoxicated with cannabis. Avoid feeding them with or mix with their food and ensure you take care of any spill over on the ground immediately.

Discard food appropriately. Try not to toss extras into the trash, where a pet or kid could get a hold of it.

A pregnant woman or nursing mother should stay clear of cannabis.

Do not consume cannabis unless you have received counsel from your physician. Cannabis can increase your susceptibility to respiratory insufficiency; compromise your immune system, affects heart function, and decrease sperm check and quality. It could exacerbate certain health illness in a sick person. To know your risk level, engage your physician.

When you eat too much Cannabis

- Relax and breathe in and out five consecutive times in a row.

- Keep in mind, cannabis does not cause death. Cannabis isn't harmful to your body. It incites awkward physical response; however, you only perceive the dread in your mind. As lethal as it feels, the circumstance is, luckily is brief.

- Lay with any of your sides, do not use your back to prevent low pulse reading and may make you feel unwell.

- To dispose chaos in your vision, close your eyes and breathe for relaxation.

- Get hold of a juice drink to raise your glucose level and make you feel more comfortable and steadier.

- Get some CBD. CBD directs THC's psychoactive impacts. Placing one or two high-CBD, low-THC tincture under the tongue could adjust the THC blast.

- Consume oranges. Citrus is a natural product richly with terrene limonene, which can help alleviate solid THC impacts. Persians endorsed it as a remedy to intoxication with cannabis in the tenth century.

- Find support by opening up to those around you that you've had an awful response and request they put an eye on you. If you ever feel your case is extraordinary, request from someone to drive you to a nearby crises center or call the emergency number. Stay away from public transport or driving yourself.

COMMON PREPARATION MISTAKES TO AVOID

You avoid the common mistakes individuals make when they cook with cannabis, regardless of whether you're new to making edibles or you've never fully taken care of business. You should pursue to amend your mistakes and keep pushing on until you achieve a delight in the world of cooking with cannabis. There are numerous innovative approaches to appreciate cannabis, and edibles are among top choices. You can make intense edibles unfailingly if you avoid the common errors.

Granulating Your Cannabis Too Fine

Some of the cannabis gourmet experts suggested the use of food or coffee processor to crush cannabis, there are persuading reasons not to. Pummeling the bud produce edibles with a verdant flavor you may not appreciate, and it can make your margarine or oil turn a dull shade of green. Rather, utilize a coarse processor and you might be looking at a perfect consistency of coarse salt.

Spending Huge Amounts of Money on Your Cooking Bud

A little goes far. Numerous beginners squander bunches of bud when they begin testing in the kitchen. When all is said in done, you should not be bothered with a tremendous measure of cannabis to make the punch you are searching for.

In contrast to smoking, you aren't simply hoping to utilize the primo bud. You can likewise extricate significant cannabinoids from shake, stems, leaves, and trim. Shake is the extra pieces at the base of your sack often known to contains a blend of a few sorts of cannabis. Business kitchens, particularly in the United States, frequently utilize blended bud for cooking, think about this choice, if you can discover it. Smoking should be done with the prime bud.

Neglecting to Add Water to Your Oil or Butter

A relatively few idealists will disclose to you this is noise, adding water to your infusion is a clever stunt. Along these lines, your margarine/oil won't consume and your cannabinoids won't debase. There is no definite measure of water to be included; your attempt is to be based on using the same quantity of oil or margarine. The water bubbles off. You can likewise observe the distinction in your "washed" finished result. It isn't as green.

Not Testing the Potency of Your Infusion Before Cooking

It should not be a Russian roulette when you prepare cannabis in the home, to test the octane, it is essential, particularly if attempting another recipe. Look at how intense your imbuement is before you commence cooking. Take a little teaspoon of your recently enriched fat as an individual portion. To check the impacts, suspend for an hour. This will assist you with deciding how solid the cluster is. Another option is to include your infusion by fixing or shower it over a recipe at the initial stage. This is an easy method to regulate the portion and measure the impacts when taken with food, and to decide to what extent it takes to kick in.

Not Knowing How to Incorporate Concentrates

For an expert to get it right with premade concentrates, it takes some time practicing. To cook with kier is relatively easy and interesting. Its fine surface breaks down in fluids and fats with ease, in some cases where a room temperature is maintained. In other to prepare hash, you need to make the necessary preparation which is dependent on the consistency, and to have a finely grounded hash, it can be placed inside a food processor.

Due to potency of concentrated cannabis compare with the customary bud, so you will require nearly less to accomplish a similar potency. This is particularly obvious with present day concentrates like waxes, oils,

Disregarding Strain Choice

In unequivocally a similar route as when you're smoking it, various strains advance various impacts, and this is in relation with the hereditary characteristics of the plant (Indica versus sativa), the mainstay here is certain cannabinoid and terpene.

The flavors and smell of a plant is linked with terpenes. As one become familiar with cannabis, studies are revealing that terpenes influence the impacts of cannabis. The impact of cannabis mixture is indicative of the associative effects of different chemical components. This is applicable to THC, CBD, terpenes similar to those seen in other plant mixture.

Utilizing Cannabis Responsibly

You ought to consistently utilize cannabis in a protected and mindful way. Similar to other medication, misuse is feasible with cannabis consumption. For no reason, you should not have the mindsets of utilizing cannabis at extraordinary levels to build the impact to a state of losing control.

There is little evidence to support physical dependence associated with cannabis consumption, some clinical experts have observed individuals experiencing addictions. It might be important to rethink and consult your doctor if you can't cope adequately with your daily living activities and when you experience low productivity and decreased efficiency.

Avoid the simultaneous consumption of cannabis when driving, working overwhelming hardware, or risky gear. Continuously know about your environmental factors and ensure you stay away from dangerous situations while sedated. Always be ready for cannabis impacts whenever you consume it and don't take it when you cannot stay put in a mindful and safe setting. It is important to have a good knowledge on how cannabis interact with different substances you might be taking, including liquor and medications.

Cannabis ought to add to your wellbeing and health, not degrade it. Comprehend your constraints and exercise watchfulness. Never permit social strain to impact your cannabis use rehearses. Know about the circumstance and figure out what measure of cannabis, assuming any, is suitable. It is your obligation to guarantee that cannabis doesn't get under the control of others, including youngsters.

If you live in a state with little or no legal protection, you should be secretive as much as possible when law enforcement agent comes around. It is never suggested to move around openly with cannabis in broad daylight, regardless of whether it is lawful in your vicinity or not. Adhere strictly to healthy protocols and it will make your experience utilizing clinical cannabis increasingly pleasant. It is dependent upon you to control the circumstance and ensure that cannabis is utilized securely.